The Nourished Pregnancy

A Self-Help Guide to Optimal Nutrition and Wellness

ROSE HARPER

TABLE OF CONTENT

Introduction

Welcome to The Nourished Pregnancy, a haven for expectant mothers and those planning to embrace the joy of motherhood. This isn't just another pregnancy guide; it's a comprehensive self-help book crafted to empower your journey to motherhood with science-backed nutrition and wellness practices.

In the unfolding chapters of The Nourished Pregnancy: A Self-Help Guide to Optimal Nutrition and Wellness, you will discover the powerful role nutrition plays in preparing your body for this wonderful life phase, and how simple yet effective wellness practices can make your pregnancy journey smoother and more fulfilling. You will find insights into how the right foods can boost your energy, enhance your mood, and promote the healthy development of your baby.

Human beings have birthed babies since time immemorial. However, modern advancements and a deeper understanding of prenatal health have shown us that it's not just about surviving pregnancy, but thriving through it. You will learn why good health and proper nutrition are imperative not only for you but also for the healthy development of your baby. From understanding essential vitamins and minerals to avoiding common nutritional pitfalls, this book covers all the essentials.

You may ask what sets this book apart from other pregnancy guides? The answer lies within these pages where ancient wisdom meets modern science to provide you with actionable information, easy-to-follow meal plans, and workouts tailored for pregnancy, and mindfulness techniques that work in harmony with your body and mind during pregnancy. The book merges tried and true nutritional practices with the latest research to offer you practical advice that you can implement in your daily life.

The author, a highly regarded expert in maternity nutrition and wellness, shares her vast knowledge and personal experiences handling various pregnancy scenarios. She pours in years of experience, love, care, and thorough research into every advice given. Her expertise lends credibility to the goldmine of information found in this guide. With qualifications in dietetics and maternal health, the author's guidance is both trustworthy and compassionate.

As you embark on this miraculous journey, let The Nourished Pregnancy be your trusted companion. Be assured that you are arming yourself with vital knowledge that will help you nourish and prepare your body optimally for one of life's most beautiful experiences. Dive into these pages, absorb the wisdom within, and step confidently onto the path of an enriched and nourished pregnancy. Embrace this guide as your partner in wellness, supporting you every step of the way towards a healthy, happy pregnancy.

Chapter 1:

Weight Gain: Nourishing Your Body

Pregnancy is a time of transformation, growth, and profound nurturing. Amidst the excitement of expecting a new life, one aspect often surrounded by confusion and anxiety is weight gain. The focus should not solely be on the numbers on the scale but rather on how nourishment can enhance not only the health of the expectant mother but also the developing baby. This chapter dives into the essential yet often misunderstood topic of weight gain during pregnancy, emphasizing the significance of healthy weight gain, providing guidelines for appropriate weight gain, and elucidating the crucial role of calorie consumption.

Here, we will explore why healthy weight gain is fundamental to a successful pregnancy and how it directly influences the development of your baby. We'll debunk common misconceptions and present evidence-based facts that underscore the importance of a balanced approach to weight gain.

Next, we will address the question that lingers in the minds of many expectant mothers: "How much weight should I gain?" Understanding that this varies based on individual factors, we will provide a comprehensive guide to recommended weight gain ranges, taking into account pre-pregnancy body mass index (BMI), multiple pregnancies, and other influencing factors. Practical tips to help you achieve and maintain this weight gain healthily will also be included.

Finally, we will go into the critical role of calories during pregnancy. Calories are not merely numbers on a nutrition label; they provide the essential energy necessary to sustain both mother and baby. We'll discuss how to balance calorie intake, ensuring you consume enough to support your pregnancy while maintaining a nutritious and balanced diet.

As you read through this chapter, you will gain valuable insights and practical advice to support a nourishing and healthy pregnancy. Let's embark on this journey to understand and embrace the importance of weight gain as a vital component of your pregnancy wellness.

The Importance of Healthy Weight Gain: Understanding the Role of Weight Gain in Pregnancy

Weight gain during pregnancy is not merely about increasing body mass; it's a multifaceted process that supports the growth and development of your baby. Gaining the right amount of weight is crucial for the health of both the mother and the child. Adequate weight gain ensures that your baby receives essential nutrients and that your body is prepared for the changes and demands of pregnancy, labor, and breastfeeding.

Healthy weight gain during pregnancy contributes to the development of the placenta, amniotic fluid, and other tissues that support your baby. It also helps build up maternal fat stores, which are essential for breastfeeding. Furthermore, appropriate weight gain can reduce the risk of pregnancy complications such as preterm birth, low birth weight, and developmental issues in the baby.

One of the common misconceptions about pregnancy weight gain is the notion that "eating for two" means consuming double the amount of food. In reality, the quality of the food you consume is far more important than the quantity. A balanced diet rich in essential nutrients supports healthy weight gain and ensures that both you and your baby are well-nourished.

Another important aspect to consider is that the rate of weight gain matters. Typically, most women gain 1-4 pounds in the first trimester and approximately 1 pound per week during the second and third trimesters. This gradual increase helps ensure that the weight gained is primarily due to the baby's growth and the necessary physiological changes in the mother's body, rather than excess fat.

Personal Stories:
Consider Sarah, who was initially anxious about gaining weight during her pregnancy. By focusing on balanced nutrition and regular check-ups, she ensured her weight gain was healthy. Sarah's story highlights how understanding the importance of weight gain can lead to a healthier and more confident pregnancy experience.

The Role of Macronutrients:
Proteins, carbohydrates, and fats all play vital roles in supporting healthy weight gain. Proteins are essential for the growth of fetal tissue, including the brain, while carbohydrates provide the necessary energy. Healthy fats are crucial for brain development and maintaining the mother's

energy levels. Examples of nutrient-rich foods include lean meats, whole grains, avocados, and nuts.

Expert Opinions:
Dr. Emily Carter, an obstetrician, emphasizes, "Healthy weight gain during pregnancy is about quality over quantity. Ensuring a balanced diet rich in nutrients supports both mother and baby and reduces the risk of complications."

Cultural Perspectives:
In many cultures, traditional practices emphasize the importance of nutrition during pregnancy. For instance, in Indian culture, there are specific dietary recommendations to ensure that both the mother and baby receive adequate nutrition, such as consuming ghee (clarified butter) for healthy fat intake.

Nutrition Tips:
First Trimester: Focus on folate-rich foods like leafy greens, beans, and citrus fruits to support early fetal development.
Second Trimester: Incorporate protein-rich foods like lean meats, dairy, and legumes to support tissue growth.
Third Trimester: Increase intake of omega-3 fatty acids found in fish and flaxseeds to support brain development.

Psychologically, healthy weight gain can also positively impact the mother's mental health. It helps in maintaining a positive body image and reduces anxiety about weight-related complications. Embracing the natural changes in your body and understanding their purpose can make the experience of pregnancy more fulfilling and less stressful.
Healthy weight gain during pregnancy is essential for supporting the physiological needs of the mother and the developmental requirements of the baby. By focusing on balanced nutrition and understanding the role of weight gain, expectant mothers can contribute to a healthier pregnancy and a better start for their babies.

Weighing In on Pregnancy: How Much Weight Should You Gain?
The question of how much weight to gain during pregnancy is one that many expectant mothers ponder. The answer varies depending on individual factors such as pre-pregnancy body mass index (BMI), the presence of multiple pregnancies (e.g., twins or triplets), and overall health. Understanding these guidelines can help ensure a healthy pregnancy for both mother and baby.

The Institute of Medicine (IOM) provides general recommendations for pregnancy weight gain based on pre-pregnancy BMI:

- ❖ Underweight (BMI < 18.5): Gain 28-40 pounds
- ❖ Normal weight (BMI 18.5-24.9): Gain 25-35 pounds
- ❖ Overweight (BMI 25-29.9): Gain 15-25 pounds
- ❖ Obese (BMI ≥ 30): Gain 11-20 pounds

These ranges are designed to optimize maternal and fetal health outcomes. For women carrying twins, the recommended weight gain is higher, typically 37-54 pounds for those with a normal pre-pregnancy BMI.

Case Studies:
Anna's Story: Anna had a normal BMI before pregnancy. She aimed to gain 25-35 pounds and focused on a balanced diet and regular exercise. Her weight gain was steady, and she felt energetic and healthy throughout her pregnancy.

Maria's Experience: Maria, who was overweight before pregnancy, worked closely with her healthcare provider to gain 15-25 pounds. By making healthier food choices and staying active, she managed her weight gain effectively and experienced a smooth pregnancy.

Expert Opinions:
Dr. Lisa Thompson, a nutritionist, advises, "It's crucial for expectant mothers to focus on gradual and steady weight gain. Sudden weight spikes or drops can indicate underlying issues that need attention. Regular consultations with healthcare providers can ensure that weight gain is on track and that both mother and baby are healthy."

Cultural Perspectives:
Different cultures have varied approaches to pregnancy nutrition. For example, in Japanese culture, there is a strong emphasis on consuming fish, rice, and vegetables to maintain a balanced diet and support healthy weight gain. These cultural practices can offer valuable insights and alternative nutritional strategies for expectant mothers.

Nutrition Tips by Trimester:
First Trimester: Emphasize folic acid intake through leafy greens, beans, and fortified cereals to support early neural development.

Second Trimester: Incorporate calcium-rich foods like dairy products, tofu, and broccoli to support bone development.

Third Trimester: Focus on iron-rich foods such as lean meats, spinach, and lentils to prevent anemia and support increased blood volume.

Factors influencing the recommended weight gain include:

Pre-pregnancy Weight: Women who are underweight may need to gain more to support the baby's growth and their own health, whereas women who are overweight or obese may need to gain less to avoid complications.

Multiple Pregnancies: Carrying more than one baby increases the need for additional weight gain to support the growth of multiple fetuses.

Health Conditions: Conditions such as gestational diabetes or hypertension may require specific weight management strategies.

Achieving healthy weight gain involves monitoring your progress and making adjustments as needed. Regular prenatal check-ups provide an opportunity for healthcare providers to assess your weight gain and overall health, offering personalized advice and support.

Here are some practical tips to help you achieve the recommended weight gain:

- ❖ Eat Balanced Meals: Focus on a diet that includes a variety of foods from all food groups. Ensure you are getting enough protein, healthy fats, carbohydrates, vitamins, and minerals.
- ❖ Stay Hydrated: Drink plenty of water throughout the day to support overall health and prevent dehydration.
- ❖ Frequent, Small Meals: Eating smaller, more frequent meals can help manage hunger and maintain steady energy levels.
- ❖ Listen to Your Body: Pay attention to hunger and fullness cues, eating when you are hungry and stopping when you are satisfied.
- ❖ Avoid Empty Calories: Limit consumption of foods high in sugar and unhealthy fats, such as sugary drinks, fast food, and processed snacks.

By understanding and following these guidelines, you can ensure that your weight gain supports a healthy pregnancy. Remember that every pregnancy is unique, and it's important to work closely with your healthcare provider to tailor your approach to your individual needs.

Counting on Calories: The Role of Calories in Supporting Your Pregnancy

Calories are not just numbers on a nutrition label; they are the units of energy that fuel your body and, during pregnancy, support the growth and development of your baby. Understanding the role of calories and how to manage your intake can help ensure a healthy pregnancy.

During pregnancy, your body's energy needs increase to support the developing fetus, the growth of the placenta, and the additional physical demands placed on your body. However, this doesn't mean doubling your calorie intake. The general recommendations for additional calorie intake during pregnancy are:

- ❖ First Trimester: No additional calories are typically needed.
- ❖ Second Trimester: An additional 340 calories per day.
- ❖ Third Trimester: An additional 450 calories per day.

These additional calories should come from nutrient-dense foods that provide vitamins, minerals, and other essential nutrients. Here are some guidelines for managing your calorie intake effectively:

Personal Stories:
Consider Jane, who carefully monitored her calorie intake during her pregnancy. By focusing on nutrient-dense foods and staying active, she maintained a healthy weight gain and felt energized throughout her pregnancy. Her experience underscores the importance of balanced nutrition and mindful eating.

Expert Opinions:
Nutritionist Dr. Michael Lee emphasizes, "While it's important to ensure adequate calorie intake during pregnancy, the focus should be on the quality of those calories. Nutrient-rich foods support both the mother's health and the baby's development, making every calorie count."

Cultural Perspectives:
In Mediterranean cultures, the diet during pregnancy often includes plenty of fresh vegetables, fruits, whole grains, and healthy fats from olive oil and fish. This balanced approach can serve as a model for maintaining proper caloric intake while ensuring optimal nutrition.

Tips for Each Trimester:

First Trimester: Focus on small, frequent meals to combat nausea and ensure a steady intake of essential nutrients.
Second Trimester: Increase portions slightly to meet the additional caloric needs, incorporating more protein and calcium-rich foods.
Third Trimester: Add healthy snacks like nuts and seeds to meet the higher calorie requirements and provide sustained energy.
Choose Nutrient-Dense Foods: Focus on whole grains, lean proteins, fruits, vegetables, and healthy fats. These foods provide the necessary nutrients without excessive calories.
Avoid Empty Calories: Limit foods and drinks high in added sugars and unhealthy fats, which offer little nutritional value.
Mindful Eating: Practice mindful eating by paying attention to hunger and fullness cues, and savoring your meals to avoid overeating.
Balanced Meals: Ensure each meal contains a balance of macronutrients (carbohydrates, proteins, and fats) to maintain steady energy levels.

In addition to managing calorie intake, the quality of the calories consumed is crucial. Here are some examples of nutrient-dense foods that can help meet your increased calorie needs:
Fruits and Vegetables: Rich in vitamins, minerals, and fiber. Examples include berries, oranges, spinach, and broccoli.
Whole Grains: Provide essential carbohydrates and fiber. Examples include oatmeal, brown rice, and whole wheat bread.
Lean Proteins: Important for the growth and repair of tissues. Examples include chicken, fish, beans, and tofu.
Healthy Fats: Essential for brain development and hormone production. Examples include avocados, nuts, seeds, and olive oil.
It's also important to note that calorie needs can vary based on individual factors such as activity level, metabolism, and overall health. Regular check-ups with your healthcare provider can help monitor your progress and make adjustments as needed.

Understanding and managing your calorie intake is a vital part of supporting a healthy pregnancy. By focusing on nutrient-dense foods and following the recommended guidelines, you can ensure that both you and your baby receive the energy and nutrients needed for a healthy and successful pregnancy journey.

Chapter 2:

The Nutrition Foundation

Welcome to Chapter 2 of "The Nourished Pregnancy: A Self-Help Guide to Optimal Nutrition and Wellness." This chapter, titled "The Nutrition Foundation," is dedicated to exploring the critical role that nutrition plays during pregnancy. Proper nutrition is the cornerstone of a healthy pregnancy, supporting both the mother's well-being and the baby's development. During these nine months, your body undergoes significant changes and requires additional nutrients to meet the needs of your growing baby. Understanding the importance of a balanced diet and the role of essential nutrients can help ensure a smooth and healthy pregnancy journey.

In this chapter, we will delve into four fundamental nutrients that form the bedrock of pregnancy nutrition: carbohydrates, fiber, protein, and healthy fats. Each of these nutrients plays a unique and vital role in supporting your body and your baby's development.

First, we will explore Carbohydrates: The Energy Source. Carbohydrates are the primary fuel for your body, providing the energy needed to support daily activities and the growing demands of pregnancy. We will discuss the differences between simple and complex carbohydrates, their sources, and recommended intake levels to keep your energy levels steady and your baby thriving.

Next, we will examine Fiber: Unlocking Optimal Digestion. Fiber is essential for maintaining healthy digestion during pregnancy, helping to prevent common issues such as constipation and regulating blood sugar levels. We will highlight fiber-rich foods that are beneficial for expectant mothers and provide practical tips for incorporating more fiber into your diet.

Following that, we will focus on Protein: Building Blocks for Baby. Protein is crucial for the growth and development of your baby, especially in forming muscles, tissues, and vital organs. We will provide guidance on the types of proteins that are most beneficial, whether from animal or plant sources, and the appropriate quantity needed during pregnancy.

Finally, we will cover Healthy Fats: Essential for Growth. Contrary to popular belief, certain fats are beneficial and necessary for both mother and baby. Healthy fats, such as omega-3 fatty acids, play a significant role in brain development and overall growth. We will discuss the importance of these fats, their sources, and how to include them in your diet.

By the end of this chapter, you will have a comprehensive understanding of these essential nutrients and practical strategies to incorporate them into your daily diet. Let's embark on this nourishing journey together, ensuring you and your baby receive the best possible nutrition.

Carbohydrates: The Energy Source

Carbohydrates are an indispensable part of a pregnant woman's diet, serving as the primary source of energy for both the mother and the developing baby. They provide the fuel necessary for everyday activities and the additional metabolic demands of pregnancy. Ensuring adequate carbohydrate intake helps maintain energy levels, supports fetal growth, and contributes to the overall well-being of the expectant mother.

Carbohydrates can be categorized into two main types: simple and complex.

Simple carbohydrates are found in foods such as fruits, milk, and sugar. They are quickly digested and provide a rapid source of energy. However, relying too heavily on simple carbohydrates, especially those from processed foods and sweets, can lead to energy spikes and crashes.

Complex carbohydrates are found in whole grains, legumes, vegetables, and certain fruits. They are digested more slowly, providing a steady release of energy. Complex carbohydrates are also rich in fiber, vitamins, and minerals, making them a healthier choice.

To ensure you are getting the right kind of carbohydrates, focus on incorporating a variety of whole foods into your diet, such as whole grains (brown rice, quinoa, oats, whole wheat bread, and barley), legumes (lentils, chickpeas, black beans, and peas), vegetables (sweet potatoes, carrots, broccoli, and leafy greens), and fruits (apples, bananas, berries, and oranges).

The recommended daily intake of carbohydrates during pregnancy is about 175 grams. This amount ensures that both the mother and the baby have enough energy to support daily functions and developmental needs. It's important to distribute carbohydrate intake evenly throughout the day to maintain stable blood sugar levels and prevent energy dips.

Carbohydrates are a vital component of a healthy pregnancy diet. By understanding the different types of carbohydrates and their sources, expectant mothers can make informed choices to support their energy needs and promote the healthy development of their babies.

Carbohydrates are paramount to a pregnant woman's diet as they act as the primary fuel for the body and mind. They support the increased energy requirements during pregnancy and play a crucial role in fetal development. Simple carbohydrates, found in foods like fruits and milk, provide quick energy but should be consumed in moderation. Complex carbohydrates, such as whole grains, vegetables, and legumes, offer sustained energy and additional nutrients essential for both mother and baby.

Ensuring adequate carbohydrate intake is vital for maintaining stable energy levels. The recommended daily intake for pregnant women is around 175 grams. This can be achieved by including a variety of carbohydrate-rich foods in your diet. Whole grains like brown rice, quinoa, and whole wheat bread are excellent sources of complex carbohydrates. Fruits like apples, bananas, and berries provide simple carbohydrates along with essential vitamins and minerals.

To incorporate more carbohydrates into your diet, consider starting your day with a high-fiber breakfast such as oatmeal topped with fruits and nuts. Include a variety of vegetables in every meal, and opt for whole grain versions of pasta, bread, and rice. Snacks like whole grain crackers, fruit with yogurt, or a small bowl of oatmeal can help maintain your energy levels throughout the day. Reducing intake of refined sugars and opting for natural sources like fruits can also help manage blood sugar levels.

Carbohydrates are a vital component of a healthy pregnancy diet. By understanding the different types of carbohydrates and their sources, expectant mothers can make informed choices to support their energy needs and promote the healthy development of their babies.

<u>**Fiber: Unlocking Optimal Digestion**</u>

Fiber, though often overlooked, plays a crucial role in maintaining optimal health during pregnancy. It is essential for supporting healthy digestion, preventing common issues like constipation, and regulating blood sugar levels. By incorporating fiber-rich foods into your diet, you can ensure smoother digestion and overall better health for both you and your baby.

Fiber is broadly classified into two types: soluble and insoluble. Soluble fiber dissolves in water to form a gel-like substance and helps lower blood cholesterol and glucose levels. Sources of soluble fiber include oats, barley, fruits like apples and oranges, and legumes. Insoluble fiber does not dissolve in water and adds bulk to the stool, aiding in the movement of material through the digestive system. Sources include whole grains, nuts, beans, and vegetables such as cauliflower and green beans.

Pregnant women should aim to consume about 25-30 grams of fiber daily. This can be achieved by including a variety of fiber-rich foods in your diet. Whole grains, such as brown rice, quinoa, whole wheat pasta, and whole grain bread, are excellent sources of fiber. Fruits like berries, apples, pears, and bananas provide fiber along with essential vitamins and minerals. Vegetables, including broccoli, carrots, sweet potatoes, and spinach, are also high in fiber and should be included in every meal. Legumes, such as lentils, black beans, chickpeas, and peas, offer both soluble and insoluble fiber. Nuts and seeds, like almonds, chia seeds, flaxseeds, and sunflower seeds, are convenient, nutrient-dense options.

To ensure you're getting enough fiber in your diet, start your day with a high-fiber breakfast such as oatmeal topped with fruits and nuts or a smoothie with spinach and chia seeds. Include a variety of vegetables in your meals, aiming for a colorful plate to ensure a range of nutrients and fiber. Choose fiber-rich snacks like raw veggies with hummus, a piece of fruit, or a handful of nuts. Replace refined grains with whole grains in your diet by opting for whole grain bread, brown rice, and whole wheat pasta. Drink plenty of water to help fiber move through your digestive system effectively.

Fiber is essential for maintaining digestive health during pregnancy. It helps prevent constipation, regulates blood sugar levels, supports heart health, and aids in weight management. Including a variety of fiber-rich foods in your diet can help ensure smoother digestion and overall better health for both you and your baby.

<u>**Protein: Building Blocks for Baby**</u>

Protein is crucial for the growth and development of your baby, especially in forming muscles, tissues, and vital organs. During pregnancy, the demand for protein increases to support the rapid growth and development of the fetus. Protein is also essential for maintaining the mother's muscle mass and supporting the production of essential hormones and enzymes.

The recommended daily intake of protein during pregnancy is about 75-100 grams. This amount can vary depending on the individual's weight, activity level, and stage of pregnancy. It's important to include a variety of protein sources in your diet to ensure you are getting all the essential amino acids needed for both you and your baby.

There are two main types of protein: animal-based and plant-based. Animal-based proteins, such as meat, poultry, fish, eggs, and dairy products, provide complete proteins, meaning they contain all the essential amino acids. Plant-based proteins, such as beans, lentils, tofu, nuts, and seeds, can also provide all the essential amino acids when consumed in a varied diet.

To ensure you are getting enough protein, include a variety of protein-rich foods in your diet. For breakfast, consider options like Greek yogurt with nuts and fruit, scrambled eggs with vegetables, or a smoothie with protein powder and spinach. For lunch and dinner, incorporate lean meats like chicken or turkey, fish, tofu, beans, or lentils into your meals. Snack on protein-rich foods like hummus with veggies, a handful of nuts, or a hard-boiled egg.

Protein is essential for the growth and development of your baby, especially in forming muscles, tissues, and vital organs. During pregnancy, the demand for protein increases to support the rapid growth and development of the fetus. Protein is also essential for maintaining the mother's muscle mass and supporting the production of essential hormones and enzymes.

The recommended daily intake of protein during pregnancy is about 75-100 grams. This amount can vary depending on the individual's weight, activity level, and stage of pregnancy. It's important to include a variety of protein sources in your diet to ensure you are getting all the essential amino acids needed for both you and your baby.

There are two main types of protein: animal-based and plant-based. Animal-based proteins, such as meat, poultry, fish, eggs, and dairy products, provide complete proteins, meaning they contain all the essential amino acids. Plant-based proteins, such as beans, lentils, tofu, nuts, and seeds, can also provide all the essential amino acids when consumed in a varied diet.

To ensure you are getting enough protein, include a variety of protein-rich foods in your diet. For breakfast, consider options like Greek yogurt with nuts and fruit, scrambled eggs with vegetables, or a smoothie with protein powder and spinach. For lunch and dinner, incorporate lean meats like chicken or turkey, fish, tofu, beans, or lentils into your meals. Snack on protein-rich foods like hummus with veggies, a handful of nuts, or a hard-boiled egg.

Including a variety of protein sources in your diet will help ensure you and your baby are getting the necessary nutrients for healthy growth and development. Protein is essential for the formation of muscles, tissues, and vital organs, making it a critical component of a healthy pregnancy diet.

Healthy Fats: Essential for Growth

Contrary to popular belief, certain fats are beneficial and necessary for both mother and baby during pregnancy. Healthy fats, such as omega-3 fatty acids, play a significant role in brain development and overall growth. Including a variety of healthy fats in your diet can support your baby's development and contribute to your overall health.

Healthy fats can be categorized into three main types: monounsaturated fats, polyunsaturated fats, and omega-3 fatty acids.

Monounsaturated fats are found in foods such as avocados, nuts, seeds, and olive oil. These fats help improve heart health by reducing bad cholesterol levels and providing essential nutrients.

Polyunsaturated fats are found in foods like fatty fish (such as salmon and sardines), flaxseeds, chia seeds, and walnuts. These fats include omega-3 and omega-6 fatty acids, which are essential for brain development and overall growth.

Omega-3 fatty acids, a type of polyunsaturated fat, are particularly important during pregnancy. They play a crucial role in the development of the baby's brain and eyes. Sources of omega-3 fatty acids include fatty fish, flaxseeds, chia seeds, walnuts, and algae-based supplements.

The recommended daily intake of healthy fats during pregnancy varies, but it is generally advised to include a moderate amount of fats in your diet, focusing on sources of monounsaturated and polyunsaturated fats. Aiming for about 20-35% of your daily caloric intake from healthy fats can help ensure you are getting the necessary nutrients.

To incorporate healthy fats into your diet, consider adding avocado slices to your salads and sandwiches, using olive oil for cooking, and including a handful of nuts or seeds in your snacks. Fatty fish like salmon can be included in your meals a couple of times a week, and flaxseeds or chia seeds can be added to smoothies, yogurt, or oatmeal.

Including a variety of healthy fats in your diet can support your baby's development and contribute to your overall health. Healthy fats, such as omega-3 fatty acids, play a significant role in brain development and overall growth. By incorporating sources of monounsaturated and polyunsaturated fats into your daily meals, you can ensure you and your baby receive the essential nutrients needed for optimal health.

Contrary to popular belief, certain fats are beneficial and necessary for both mother and baby during pregnancy. Healthy fats, such as omega-3 fatty acids, play a significant role in brain development and overall growth. Including a variety of healthy fats in your diet can support your baby's development and contribute to your overall health.

Healthy fats can be categorized into three main types: monounsaturated fats, polyunsaturated fats, and omega-3 fatty acids.

Monounsaturated fats are found in foods such as avocados, nuts, seeds, and olive oil. These fats help improve heart health by reducing bad cholesterol levels and providing essential nutrients.

Polyunsaturated fats are found in foods like fatty fish (such as salmon and sardines), flaxseeds, chia seeds, and walnuts. These fats include omega-3 and omega-6 fatty acids, which are essential for brain development and overall growth.

Omega-3 fatty acids, a type of polyunsaturated fat, are particularly important during pregnancy. They play a crucial role in the development of the baby's brain and eyes. Sources of omega-3 fatty acids include fatty fish, flaxseeds, chia seeds, walnuts, and algae-based supplements.

The recommended daily intake of healthy fats during pregnancy varies, but it is generally advised to include a moderate amount of fats in your diet, focusing on sources of monounsaturated and polyunsaturated fats. Aiming for about 20-35% of your daily caloric intake from healthy fats can help ensure you are getting the necessary nutrients.

To incorporate healthy fats into your diet, consider adding avocado slices to your salads and sandwiches, using olive oil for cooking, and including a handful of nuts or seeds in your snacks. Fatty fish like salmon can be included in your meals a couple of times a week, and flaxseeds or chia seeds can be added to smoothies, yogurt, or oatmeal.

Including a variety of healthy fats in your diet will help ensure you and your baby are getting the necessary nutrients for healthy growth and development. Healthy fats, such as omega-3 fatty acids, play a significant role in brain development and overall growth. By incorporating sources of monounsaturated and polyunsaturated fats into your daily meals, you can ensure you and your baby receive the essential nutrients needed for optimal health.

Chapter 3:

Vitamins and Minerals: The Essential Team

Pregnancy is a transformative journey that demands a keen focus on nutrition to ensure the health and well-being of both mother and baby. As you embark on this remarkable path, understanding the critical role of vitamins, minerals, and supplements becomes paramount. These essential nutrients are the building blocks of a healthy pregnancy, supporting everything from fetal development to maternal energy levels. This chapter aims to provide a comprehensive guide to the vitamins and minerals vital during pregnancy, their sources, and the importance of supplements.

You'll learn about the powerhouse vitamins like Vitamin A, which bolsters the immune system, and Vitamin D, which is crucial for bone health and mood regulation. The chapter will also delve into the significance of minerals such as Calcium for strong bones and Iron for preventing anemia. Beyond individual nutrients, we will explore the necessity of prenatal vitamins, the brain-boosting benefits of Omega-3 fatty acids, and the gut health benefits of probiotics.

Navigating the world of nutrition during pregnancy can be daunting, but this chapter is designed to empower you with knowledge and practical advice. We'll compare the benefits of obtaining nutrients from food sources versus supplements, helping you make informed decisions about your diet. Recognizing and addressing deficiencies will also be covered, along with understanding the potential risks and interactions of various supplements with other medications.

In addition to the technical aspects of nutrition, we'll provide guidance on creating personalized nutrition plans tailored to your individual needs. You'll also find tips for managing common pregnancy-related nutrition concerns, such as morning sickness and cravings. By the end of this chapter, you will be equipped with the information and confidence to make the best nutritional choices for you and your baby during this extraordinary time.

<u>Vital Vitamins and Minerals</u>

Vitamin A: Essential for Vision and Immune Function
Vitamin A plays a crucial role in maintaining healthy vision, immune function, and cell growth.
During pregnancy, it is particularly important for fetal development, especially for the heart,
lungs, kidneys, and eyes. It also helps ensure that the immune system is functioning optimally,
protecting both the mother and baby from infections.
Sources of Vitamin A include both animal and plant-based foods. Retinoids, the active form of
Vitamin A, are found in animal products such as liver, fish, and dairy. Carotenoids, which are
converted into Vitamin A in the body, are abundant in colorful fruits and vegetables like carrots,
sweet potatoes, and spinach.

While Vitamin A is vital, it's important to monitor intake, especially during pregnancy.
Excessive amounts can be harmful and have been associated with birth defects. The
recommended daily allowance (RDA) for pregnant women is 770 micrograms, and it's essential
to avoid supplements containing high doses of preformed Vitamin A.

Vitamin D: Supporting Bone Health and Mood Regulation
Vitamin D is another critical nutrient during pregnancy, aiding in the absorption of calcium and
promoting healthy bone development for both mother and baby. It also plays a role in immune
function and has been linked to mood regulation, helping to prevent depression and anxiety
during pregnancy and postpartum.

The primary source of Vitamin D is sunlight exposure, which triggers the synthesis of Vitamin
D in the skin. However, many people, especially those living in northern latitudes or with
limited sun exposure, may require dietary sources or supplements. Foods rich in Vitamin D
include fatty fish like salmon and mackerel, fortified milk and orange juice, and egg yolks.

Pregnant women should aim for an intake of 600 IU (15 micrograms) of Vitamin D per day.
Given the difficulty of obtaining sufficient Vitamin D from diet and sunlight alone, many
healthcare providers recommend a Vitamin D supplement during pregnancy to ensure adequate
levels.

Folic Acid: Preventing Neural Tube Defects
Folic acid, or Vitamin B9, is perhaps one of the most well-known vitamins related to pregnancy.
It is essential for the formation of the neural tube, which develops into the baby's brain and

spinal cord. Adequate folic acid intake before and during early pregnancy can significantly reduce the risk of neural tube defects such as spina bifida and anencephaly.

Leafy green vegetables, citrus fruits, beans, and fortified cereals are excellent sources of folic acid. However, due to the critical importance of this vitamin in early pregnancy, women of childbearing age are often advised to take a folic acid supplement of 400 to 800 micrograms daily, starting at least one month before conception and continuing through the first trimester.

Vitamin C: Enhancing Iron Absorption and Immune Function
Vitamin C, known for its antioxidant properties, supports the immune system, aids in the production of collagen, and enhances the absorption of iron from plant-based foods. This is particularly important during pregnancy to prevent anemia and support the increased blood volume.

Citrus fruits, strawberries, bell peppers, and broccoli are rich sources of Vitamin C. The RDA for pregnant women is 85 milligrams per day. While it's generally easy to meet this requirement through diet, Vitamin C supplements are also available if needed.

Vitamin E: Protecting Cells from Damage
Vitamin E is an antioxidant that helps protect cells from damage and supports immune function. It also plays a role in the development of the baby's organs and tissues. Nuts, seeds, spinach, and fortified cereals are good sources of Vitamin E.

The RDA for Vitamin E during pregnancy is 15 milligrams per day. It's important to avoid excessive supplementation, as high doses of Vitamin E can interfere with blood clotting and increase the risk of bleeding.

Vitamin K: Essential for Blood Clotting
Vitamin K is crucial for blood clotting, which is important during delivery to prevent excessive bleeding. It also supports bone health. Leafy green vegetables, broccoli, and Brussels sprouts are excellent sources of Vitamin K.

The RDA for pregnant women is 90 micrograms per day. Most people can meet this requirement through a balanced diet, but supplements are available if needed.

Mighty Minerals

Calcium: Building Strong Bones and Teeth
Calcium is an essential mineral for the development of strong bones and teeth in the growing baby. It also supports muscle function, nerve signaling, and the release of hormones. During pregnancy, the body increases its efficiency in absorbing calcium, but it is still crucial to ensure an adequate intake to prevent depletion of the mother's calcium stores, which could lead to weakened bones and teeth.

Dairy products such as milk, cheese, and yogurt are well-known sources of calcium. For those who are lactose intolerant or prefer non-dairy options, fortified plant-based milks (like almond, soy, or oat milk), tofu, leafy green vegetables, and calcium-fortified orange juice are excellent alternatives.

The recommended daily allowance (RDA) for calcium during pregnancy is 1,000 milligrams. Pregnant teenagers (aged 14-18) need slightly more, about 1,300 milligrams per day. If dietary intake is insufficient, a calcium supplement may be recommended by a healthcare provider. It is also important to pair calcium intake with Vitamin D to enhance absorption.

Iron: Preventing Anemia and Supporting Oxygen Transport
Iron is a vital mineral during pregnancy as it supports the increased blood volume and helps in the formation of hemoglobin, which transports oxygen to the baby and maternal tissues. Adequate iron intake prevents iron-deficiency anemia, which can cause fatigue, weakness, and increased risk of infection for the mother, and poor fetal growth and preterm delivery.

Sources of iron include red meat, poultry, fish, beans, lentils, spinach, and iron-fortified cereals. The iron from animal sources (heme iron) is more readily absorbed by the body compared to that from plant sources (non-heme iron). To improve the absorption of non-heme iron, it is beneficial to consume it with Vitamin C-rich foods like citrus fruits, tomatoes, or bell peppers.

The RDA for iron during pregnancy is 27 milligrams per day, nearly double the requirement for non-pregnant women. Given the challenges of obtaining sufficient iron from diet alone, especially for vegetarians and vegans, an iron supplement is often recommended.

Magnesium: Supporting Muscle and Nerve Function
Magnesium plays several critical roles during pregnancy, including muscle and nerve function, regulating blood sugar levels, and promoting a healthy immune system. It also helps build and repair tissues and can help alleviate leg cramps, a common discomfort during pregnancy.

Good dietary sources of magnesium include nuts and seeds, whole grains, legumes, leafy green vegetables, and fortified foods.

The RDA for magnesium during pregnancy varies by age: 350 milligrams per day for pregnant women aged 19-30, and 360 milligrams per day for those aged 31 and older. Magnesium supplements are available, but it is advisable to consult with a healthcare provider before starting any supplementation, as high doses can cause diarrhea and other digestive issues.

Zinc: Promoting Growth and Immune Function
Zinc is crucial for DNA synthesis, cell division, and protein synthesis, making it essential for the growth and development of the fetus. It also supports the immune system and helps in wound healing.

Sources of zinc include meat, shellfish, dairy products, nuts, seeds, legumes, and whole grains. Zinc from animal sources is more easily absorbed than that from plant sources.

The RDA for zinc during pregnancy is 11 milligrams per day for women aged 19 and older, and 12 milligrams per day for pregnant teenagers aged 14-18. Most women can meet this requirement through a balanced diet, but supplements can be taken if necessary.

Iodine: Supporting Thyroid Function and Brain Development
Iodine is vital for the production of thyroid hormones, which regulate metabolism, and are essential for brain development and growth in the fetus. Iodine deficiency during pregnancy can lead to serious complications such as cretinism, a condition characterized by severe physical and mental retardation.

Iodized salt, dairy products, seafood, and eggs are good sources of iodine. However, with the increased use of non-iodized salt and varying iodine content in foods, some women may require an iodine supplement.

The RDA for iodine during pregnancy is 220 micrograms per day. Ensuring adequate iodine intake is particularly important for pregnant women living in regions where soil and food supply have low iodine levels.

Selenium: Protecting Against Oxidative Stress
Selenium is an important antioxidant that protects cells from damage and supports thyroid function and the immune system. During pregnancy, it helps in the development of the baby's brain and reduces the risk of preeclampsia.

Sources of selenium include Brazil nuts, seafood, meat, eggs, and whole grains.

The RDA for selenium during pregnancy is 60 micrograms per day. While most people can meet their selenium needs through diet, supplements are available if required.

Copper: Forming Red Blood Cells and Supporting Iron Absorption
Copper is essential for forming red blood cells, maintaining healthy nerves and immune function, and assisting in iron absorption. It also plays a role in developing the baby's heart, blood vessels, and skeletal and nervous systems.

Good sources of copper include organ meats, shellfish, nuts, seeds, whole grains, and legumes.

The RDA for copper during pregnancy is 1,000 micrograms (1 milligram) per day. A balanced diet typically provides sufficient copper, but supplements are available if needed.

Prenatal Vitamins: The Essential Multivitamin for Pregnancy

Prenatal vitamins are specially formulated multivitamins that provide essential nutrients to support both the mother and the developing baby. They contain higher levels of certain vitamins and minerals than standard multivitamins, tailored to meet the increased nutritional needs during pregnancy.

A good prenatal vitamin typically includes folic acid, iron, calcium, vitamin D, DHA (an omega-3 fatty acid), and other essential nutrients like iodine, zinc, and vitamins A, C, and E. The exact composition can vary between brands, so it's important to choose a prenatal vitamin that suits individual nutritional needs, as recommended by a healthcare provider.

Folic acid, for instance, is crucial for preventing neural tube defects and should be taken even before conception. Iron supports the increased blood volume and helps prevent anemia. Calcium and vitamin D are important for the development of the baby's bones and teeth, while DHA supports brain and eye development.

While prenatal vitamins can help fill nutritional gaps, they should not replace a balanced diet. The goal is to supplement the diet, not substitute it. It's recommended to start taking prenatal vitamins before conception and continue throughout the pregnancy and breastfeeding period.

Omega-3 Fatty Acids: Supporting Brain and Eye Development
Omega-3 fatty acids, particularly DHA (docosahexaenoic acid) and EPA (eicosapentaenoic acid), are essential for the development of the baby's brain and eyes. They also help reduce the risk of preterm birth and support the mother's mental health by potentially lowering the risk of postpartum depression.

These fatty acids are found in fatty fish like salmon, mackerel, and sardines, as well as in flaxseeds, chia seeds, walnuts, and algae-based supplements. However, due to concerns about mercury content in certain fish, many pregnant women turn to omega-3 supplements.

The recommended intake of DHA and EPA during pregnancy is about 200-300 milligrams per day. Fish oil supplements are a common source, but it's important to choose high-quality, purified products to avoid contaminants. Algae-based supplements are a good plant-based alternative.

Probiotics: Enhancing Gut Health
Probiotics are beneficial bacteria that support a healthy digestive system and enhance the immune system. During pregnancy, they can help manage digestive issues like constipation and diarrhea, reduce the risk of gestational diabetes, and potentially lower the incidence of allergies in the baby.

Probiotics are found in fermented foods such as yogurt, kefir, sauerkraut, kimchi, and kombucha. Supplements are also available in various forms, including capsules, powders, and liquids.

There is no specific recommended daily allowance for probiotics, as the optimal dosage can vary. It's advisable to consult a healthcare provider to determine the right type and amount of probiotic supplement during pregnancy.

Vitamin D Supplements: Ensuring Adequate Levels
Vitamin D is crucial for calcium absorption and bone health. It also plays a role in immune function and cell division. During pregnancy, adequate vitamin D levels are necessary to support the skeletal development of the baby and prevent complications like preeclampsia and low birth weight.

Sunlight exposure is a primary source of vitamin D, but factors such as geographic location, skin pigmentation, and sunscreen use can limit synthesis. Dietary sources include fatty fish, fortified dairy products, and egg yolks, but it can be challenging to meet the needs through diet alone.

The RDA for vitamin D during pregnancy is 600 IU (15 micrograms) per day, but some experts recommend higher doses, especially for those with limited sun exposure. Vitamin D3 supplements are often preferred for their effectiveness in raising blood levels of vitamin D.

Iron Supplements: Preventing Anemia
Iron supplements are commonly recommended during pregnancy to support the increased blood volume and prevent iron-deficiency anemia. Anemia during pregnancy can lead to fatigue, weakness, and increased susceptibility to infections, and it can affect the baby's growth and development.

Iron supplements come in various forms, including ferrous sulfate, ferrous gluconate, and ferrous fumarate. The choice of supplement and dosage depends on the individual's iron levels, as determined by blood tests. Typically, 27 milligrams of iron per day is recommended, which is often included in prenatal vitamins.

It's important to take iron supplements with vitamin C to enhance absorption and avoid taking them with calcium-rich foods or supplements, which can inhibit absorption. Side effects of iron supplements may include constipation and stomach upset, so it's advisable to discuss any concerns with a healthcare provider.

Calcium Supplements: Building Strong Bones
Calcium supplements may be necessary for those who cannot meet their calcium needs through diet alone. Adequate calcium intake is essential for the development of the baby's bones and teeth and to prevent the mother's bone density loss.

Calcium carbonate and calcium citrate are common forms of calcium supplements. Calcium carbonate requires stomach acid for absorption and is best taken with food, while calcium citrate is absorbed well on an empty stomach and is a better option for those with acid reflux.

The RDA for calcium during pregnancy is 1,000 milligrams per day. It's important not to exceed the upper limit of 2,500 milligrams per day to avoid potential adverse effects like kidney stones.

The Importance of Food Sources

Whole foods are the best source of vitamins and minerals because they provide a complex mix of nutrients and other beneficial compounds, such as fiber and antioxidants that are not found in supplements. Foods like fruits, vegetables, whole grains, lean proteins, and dairy products offer a balance of nutrients that work synergistically to support overall health and wellness.

During pregnancy, a diet rich in whole foods can help ensure that you and your baby receive the necessary nutrients for growth and development. For instance, leafy green vegetables like spinach and kale are excellent sources of folate, which is critical for preventing neural tube defects. Dairy products, fortified plant-based milks, and certain fish like salmon provide calcium and vitamin D for bone health. Lean meats, beans, and lentils offer iron, which is essential for preventing anemia and supporting increased blood volume.

Advantages of Whole Foods

Nutrient Density: Whole foods are nutrient-dense, meaning they provide a high amount of vitamins and minerals relative to their calorie content. This is important for meeting the increased nutritional needs during pregnancy without excessive calorie intake.

Bioavailability: Nutrients in whole foods are often more bioavailable, meaning they are more easily absorbed and utilized by the body. For example, the iron in meat (heme iron) is more readily absorbed than the iron in plant-based foods (non-heme iron).

Additional Health Benefits: Whole foods contain other beneficial compounds like antioxidants, phytochemicals, and fiber, which can support overall health. Antioxidants help protect cells from damage, phytochemicals have various health-promoting properties, and fiber supports digestive health and can help prevent constipation, a common issue during pregnancy.

When Are Supplements Necessary?

Despite the advantages of whole foods, there are circumstances where supplements become necessary during pregnancy. Supplements can help fill nutritional gaps that may arise due to various factors such as dietary restrictions, morning sickness, or increased nutritional demands.

Folic Acid: Folic acid is crucial for preventing neural tube defects, and it's difficult to obtain sufficient amounts from food alone. Therefore, supplementation is recommended before conception and during early pregnancy.

Iron: The increased blood volume during pregnancy raises the need for iron. While iron-rich foods are beneficial, many women still require iron supplements to prevent anemia.

Vitamin D: Limited sun exposure, especially in certain geographic locations or during winter months, can make it challenging to obtain adequate vitamin D from sunlight and food sources alone. Supplements can help maintain optimal levels.

Calcium: While dairy products and fortified foods are good sources of calcium, some women may not consume enough of these foods, especially if they are lactose intolerant or follow a vegan diet. Supplements can help meet the required intake.

Omega-3 Fatty Acids: Although fatty fish is an excellent source of omega-3 fatty acids, concerns about mercury contamination may limit consumption. Omega-3 supplements, particularly those derived from algae, can provide a safer alternative.

Balancing Food and Supplements

Achieving a balance between obtaining nutrients from whole foods and using supplements when necessary is key to a healthy pregnancy. Here are some guidelines for balancing both:

Prioritize Whole Foods: Aim to meet most of your nutritional needs through a varied diet that includes a wide range of fruits, vegetables, whole grains, lean proteins, and dairy or fortified plant-based alternatives.

Supplement Wisely: Use supplements to fill specific gaps identified by your healthcare provider. This may include prenatal vitamins, iron, folic acid, vitamin D, omega-3 fatty acids, and calcium.

Consult with Healthcare Providers: Regular check-ups and consultations with your healthcare provider can help monitor your nutritional status and adjust your supplement regimen as needed.

Avoid Over-Supplementation: Excessive intake of certain vitamins and minerals can be harmful. Follow the recommended dosages and avoid taking multiple supplements that provide the same nutrient.

Combine with a Healthy Lifestyle: A balanced diet combined with other healthy lifestyle practices, such as regular physical activity, adequate hydration, and sufficient sleep, contributes to overall wellness during pregnancy.

Recognizing Deficiencies and Insufficiencies

During pregnancy, it's essential to recognize the signs of nutrient deficiencies and insufficiencies to address them promptly. Common deficiencies during pregnancy include iron, vitamin D, and folate, each presenting specific symptoms and requiring targeted interventions. For Example

Iron Deficiency:

Symptoms: Fatigue, weakness, shortness of breath, pale skin, dizziness, and headaches.
Intervention: Incorporate iron-rich foods such as lean meats, beans, lentils, spinach, and fortified cereals. Iron supplements may be necessary as advised by a healthcare provider.
Vitamin D Deficiency:

Symptoms: Bone pain, muscle weakness, fatigue, and an increased risk of infections.
Intervention: Increase sun exposure, consume vitamin D-rich foods like fatty fish, fortified dairy products, and consider vitamin D supplements.
Folate Deficiency:

Symptoms: Fatigue, mouth sores, tongue swelling, and growth problems in the baby.
Intervention: Consume folate-rich foods like leafy greens, legumes, and citrus fruits. Supplement with folic acid as recommended by a healthcare provider.
Recognizing these symptoms and taking appropriate actions can help maintain optimal health for both mother and baby during pregnancy.

Understanding Nutrient Deficiencies and Insufficiencies

Nutrient deficiencies and insufficiencies can have significant impacts on maternal and fetal health during pregnancy. A deficiency occurs when the intake or absorption of a nutrient is inadequate to meet the body's needs, leading to clinical symptoms and health problems. Insufficiency, on the other hand, refers to suboptimal levels that may not cause overt symptoms but can still affect overall health and development.

During pregnancy, the body's demand for certain nutrients increases to support the growth and development of the baby as well as the mother's own health. Identifying and addressing nutrient deficiencies and insufficiencies is crucial for preventing complications and ensuring a healthy pregnancy outcome.

Common Nutrient Deficiencies in Pregnancy

Iron Deficiency

- ❖ Importance: Iron is essential for producing hemoglobin, the protein in red blood cells that carries oxygen to the body's tissues. During pregnancy, blood volume increases significantly, raising the demand for iron.
- ❖ Symptoms: Fatigue, weakness, shortness of breath, pale skin, dizziness, and headaches are common symptoms of iron deficiency anemia.
- ❖ Sources: Lean meats, poultry, fish, beans, lentils, spinach, and iron-fortified cereals are excellent dietary sources of iron.
- ❖ Intervention: Iron supplements may be necessary if dietary intake is insufficient. It is important to take iron supplements as advised by a healthcare provider, as excessive iron can cause gastrointestinal issues and other problems.

Vitamin D Deficiency

- ❖ Importance: Vitamin D is crucial for calcium absorption and bone health. It also plays a role in immune function and inflammation regulation.
- ❖ Symptoms: Bone pain, muscle weakness, fatigue, and an increased risk of infections can indicate vitamin D deficiency.
- ❖ Sources: Fatty fish (such as salmon and mackerel), fortified dairy products, and exposure to sunlight are primary sources of vitamin D.
- ❖ Intervention: Vitamin D supplements may be necessary, especially in individuals with limited sun exposure or dietary intake.

Folate (Vitamin B9) Deficiency

- ❖ Importance: Folate is vital for DNA synthesis, cell division, and preventing neural tube defects in the developing fetus.
- ❖ Symptoms: Fatigue, mouth sores, tongue swelling, and growth problems in the baby can signal folate deficiency.
- ❖ Sources: Leafy green vegetables, legumes, nuts, and fortified cereals are rich in folate.

❖ Intervention: Folic acid supplements are recommended before conception and during early pregnancy to ensure adequate levels.

Calcium Deficiency

❖ Importance: Calcium is necessary for the development of the baby's bones and teeth, as well as for maintaining the mother's bone health.
❖ Symptoms: Muscle cramps, tooth decay, and an increased risk of osteoporosis can result from calcium deficiency.
❖ Sources: Dairy products, fortified plant-based milks, leafy green vegetables, and tofu are good sources of calcium.
❖ Intervention: Calcium supplements may be recommended for those who do not consume enough calcium-rich foods.

Iodine Deficiency

❖ Importance: Iodine is critical for thyroid function, which regulates metabolism and is essential for fetal brain development.
❖ Symptoms: Goiter (enlarged thyroid gland), fatigue, weight gain, and developmental delays in the baby can occur due to iodine deficiency.
❖ Sources: Iodized salt, seafood, dairy products, and eggs provide iodine.
❖ Intervention: Iodine supplements may be necessary for those with dietary restrictions or living in areas with low iodine soil content.

Identifying Deficiencies and Insufficiencies

Regular prenatal check-ups include blood tests to monitor levels of essential nutrients. These tests help identify any deficiencies or insufficiencies early on, allowing for timely intervention. It's important for pregnant women to attend all scheduled appointments and follow their healthcare provider's recommendations.

Preventing Deficiencies

Balanced Diet: A varied diet that includes a wide range of nutrient-dense foods can help prevent deficiencies. Emphasize fruits, vegetables, whole grains, lean proteins, and dairy or fortified alternatives.

Prenatal Vitamins: Prenatal vitamins are specifically formulated to meet the increased nutritional needs of pregnancy. They typically include folic acid, iron, calcium, and other essential vitamins and minerals.

Regular Monitoring: Regular blood tests and check-ups with a healthcare provider can help monitor nutrient levels and address any deficiencies promptly.

Education and Awareness: Understanding the importance of nutrition during pregnancy and recognizing the signs of deficiencies can empower women to take proactive steps in maintaining their health and the health of their baby.

Risks and Interactions

Excessive intake of certain vitamins and minerals can be harmful. For example, too much vitamin A can cause birth defects, while excessive iron can lead to gastrointestinal issues and oxidative stress. It's important to follow the recommended dosages and consult with a healthcare provider before taking any supplements.

Interactions with Medications

Some nutrients can interact with medications, affecting their efficacy or causing adverse effects. For example, calcium can interfere with the absorption of certain antibiotics, while iron can interact with thyroid medications. It's essential to inform your healthcare provider about all supplements you are taking to avoid potential interactions.

Interactions and Contraindications

During pregnancy, the interaction between nutrients and medications becomes critically important. Certain nutrients can affect the absorption, metabolism, and efficacy of medications, while some drugs can interfere with nutrient absorption and utilization. Recognizing these interactions and contraindications helps ensure that both mother and baby receive the necessary nutrients without adverse effects.

Common Nutrient-Drug Interactions

Calcium and Antibiotics
- ❖ Interaction: Calcium can bind to certain antibiotics (such as tetracyclines and fluoroquinolones), reducing their absorption and effectiveness.
- ❖ Management: To prevent this interaction, it is recommended to take antibiotics at least two hours before or six hours after consuming calcium-rich foods or supplements.

Iron and Thyroid Medications
*   ❖ Interaction: Iron supplements can decrease the absorption of levothyroxine, a common thyroid medication, potentially leading to reduced efficacy and altered thyroid hormone levels.
*   ❖ Management: To minimize this interaction, it is advised to take iron supplements and thyroid medication at least four hours apart.

Folic Acid and Methotrexate
*   ❖ Interaction: Methotrexate, a medication used for certain autoimmune diseases and cancer, can interfere with folic acid metabolism, leading to a deficiency.
*   ❖ Management: Healthcare providers may prescribe folic acid supplements to counteract this interaction and prevent deficiency.

Vitamin K and Anticoagulants
*   ❖ Interaction: Vitamin K can interfere with the effectiveness of anticoagulant medications (such as warfarin) used to prevent blood clots. Vitamin K is essential for blood clotting, and its intake must be consistent to avoid fluctuations in medication efficacy.
*   ❖ Management: It is crucial to maintain a consistent intake of vitamin K from dietary sources and supplements and to regularly monitor blood clotting parameters with a healthcare provider.

Magnesium and Heart Medications
*   ❖ Interaction: Magnesium supplements can affect the absorption and efficacy of certain heart medications, such as digoxin.
*   ❖ Management: To reduce the risk of interaction, magnesium supplements should be taken at least two hours before or after heart medications.

Contraindications with Nutritional Supplements

Vitamin A
*   ❖ Risk: Excessive intake of vitamin A, particularly in the form of retinol (found in animal products and some supplements), can cause teratogenic effects, leading to birth defects.
*   ❖ Management: Pregnant women should avoid high-dose vitamin A supplements and focus on obtaining this nutrient from dietary sources like beta-carotene (found in fruits and vegetables), which is safer.

Iron Overload
  - ❖ Risk: While iron is crucial during pregnancy, excessive supplementation can lead to iron overload, causing gastrointestinal distress, oxidative stress, and damage to organs.
  - ❖ Management: It is important to follow healthcare provider recommendations regarding iron supplementation and to avoid self-prescribing high doses.

Herbal Supplements
  - ❖ Risk: Some herbal supplements can have potent pharmacological effects and may not be safe during pregnancy. For example, certain herbs like St. John's Wort can interact with medications and affect fetal development.
  - ❖ Management: Pregnant women should consult with a healthcare provider before taking any herbal supplements to ensure safety.

High-Dose Vitamin C
  - ❖ Risk: While vitamin C is essential for immune function and collagen synthesis, very high doses can lead to gastrointestinal disturbances and may increase the risk of preterm labor.
  - ❖ Management: Adhering to the recommended dietary allowance (RDA) and avoiding excessive supplementation can mitigate this risk
  .

Managing Nutrient-Drug Interactions
- Consult Healthcare Providers: Always inform your healthcare provider about all supplements and medications you are taking. This allows them to manage potential interactions and adjust dosages as needed.
- Timing of Supplements: Pay attention to the timing of supplement intake relative to medications to minimize interactions. Spacing out the consumption of conflicting substances can enhance absorption and efficacy.
- Regular Monitoring: Regular check-ups and blood tests can help monitor nutrient levels and medication efficacy, allowing for timely adjustments.
- Education and Awareness: Understanding the potential interactions and contraindications can empower pregnant women to make informed decisions about their nutrition and medication management.

Guidelines for Safe Supplementation
Follow Recommended Dosages: Adhering to the dosages recommended by healthcare providers helps prevent adverse effects and interactions.
Balanced Diet: Focus on obtaining nutrients from a varied and balanced diet, using supplements to fill specific gaps as needed.

Avoid Self-Prescription: Avoid self-prescribing high doses of supplements without consulting a healthcare provider, as this can lead to harmful interactions and side effects.

Stay Informed: Stay informed about the latest research and guidelines on nutrient interactions and contraindications during pregnancy to ensure optimal health outcomes for both mother and baby.

Personalized Nutrition Planning

Personalized nutrition planning during pregnancy is essential to meet the unique needs of each expectant mother. Every woman's body responds differently to pregnancy, and factors such as age, pre-pregnancy health status, lifestyle, and dietary preferences influence nutritional requirements. A personalized approach ensures that both the mother and baby receive optimal nourishment, promoting healthy development and preventing complications.

Assessing Individual Nutritional Needs

Pre-Pregnancy Health Status

Importance: Understanding a woman's health status before pregnancy helps identify potential nutritional gaps and areas needing attention. Conditions such as anemia, diabetes, or hypertension can significantly influence dietary needs.

Action: Conduct a thorough health assessment, including medical history, blood tests, and dietary habits, to identify specific nutritional requirements.

Age and Physiological Factors

Importance: Age and physiological factors like body weight, height, and metabolic rate affect nutrient needs. For example, younger women and teenagers may have higher nutritional demands due to ongoing growth and development.

Action: Tailor nutrition plans based on age and individual physiology, ensuring adequate intake of critical nutrients like calcium, iron, and folic acid.

Lifestyle and Activity Level

Importance: A woman's lifestyle, including her physical activity level and occupational demands, impacts her caloric and nutrient requirements. Active women may require more calories and protein to support both pregnancy and their activity level.

Action: Adjust caloric intake and nutrient distribution based on activity levels, ensuring balanced energy and nutrient supply without excessive weight gain.

Dietary Preferences and Restrictions

Importance: Dietary preferences, including vegetarianism, veganism, or food allergies, affect nutrient intake. Ensuring these preferences are met without compromising essential nutrient requirements is crucial.

Action: Create meal plans that honor dietary preferences and restrictions while incorporating nutrient-dense alternatives to meet nutritional needs.

Steps to Develop a Personalized Nutrition Plan

Nutritional Assessment and Goal Setting

Initial Assessment: Begin with a comprehensive nutritional assessment, including a detailed dietary history, lifestyle evaluation, and laboratory tests to determine baseline nutritional status.

Set Goals: Collaborate with the expectant mother to set realistic and achievable nutritional goals based on her health status, lifestyle, and preferences.

Designing a Balanced Meal Plan

Macronutrient Distribution: Ensure an appropriate balance of macronutrients (carbohydrates, proteins, and fats) tailored to the individual's caloric needs and activity level. For example, emphasize complex carbohydrates for sustained energy, lean proteins for tissue repair and growth, and healthy fats for brain development.

Micronutrient Focus: Highlight key micronutrients critical during pregnancy, such as folic acid, iron, calcium, vitamin D, and omega-3 fatty acids. Incorporate a variety of food sources rich in these nutrients.

Incorporating Nutrient-Rich Foods

Whole Foods: Emphasize whole, minimally processed foods such as fruits, vegetables, whole grains, lean proteins, and healthy fats. These provide essential vitamins, minerals, and antioxidants.

Variety and Moderation: Encourage variety in the diet to cover a broad spectrum of nutrients and prevent deficiencies. Practice moderation to maintain a balanced intake without excess.

Supplementation Guidance

Supplement Needs: Identify any nutritional gaps that cannot be met through diet alone and recommend appropriate supplements. For instance, prenatal vitamins, iron supplements, or omega-3 fatty acids may be necessary.

Dosage and Timing: Provide clear instructions on supplement dosage and timing to maximize absorption and efficacy. For example, taking iron supplements with vitamin C enhances absorption, while avoiding calcium-rich foods at the same time.

Monitoring and Adjusting the Plan

Regular Check-Ins: Schedule regular follow-up appointments to monitor progress, assess nutritional status, and make necessary adjustments to the meal plan and supplements.

Feedback and Adaptation: Encourage feedback from the expectant mother regarding her dietary preferences, any challenges faced, and overall wellbeing. Adapt the plan as needed to ensure it remains practical and effective.

Tools and Resources for Personalized Nutrition Planning

Food Diaries and Tracking Apps

Utility: Using food diaries or nutrition tracking apps helps monitor daily intake, identify patterns, and ensure adherence to the nutrition plan.

Examples: MyFitnessPal, Cronometer, and Pregnancy+ are popular apps that provide detailed nutrient tracking and meal planning support.

Educational Materials and Recipes

Professional Support

Importance: Working with healthcare professionals, such as registered dietitians, nutritionists, and obstetricians, ensures a comprehensive and evidence-based approach to personalized nutrition planning.

Collaboration: Encourage collaborative care, where dietitians and healthcare providers work together to support the expectant mother's nutritional needs and overall health.

Empowering Expectant Mothers with Nutrition Knowledge

Nutritional Education

Workshops and Classes: Offer workshops and classes focused on prenatal nutrition, teaching expectant mothers about nutrient requirements, healthy food choices, and meal planning.

Online Resources: Utilize online platforms, webinars, and social media to share educational content, tips, and resources on prenatal nutrition.

Community Support Groups

Peer Support: Establish community support groups where pregnant women can share experiences, exchange recipes, and offer mutual encouragement and support.

Mentorship: Pair expectant mothers with experienced mentors who can provide guidance and practical advice on maintaining a healthy diet during pregnancy.

Personalized nutrition planning is a dynamic and individualized approach to ensuring optimal health and wellness during pregnancy. By assessing individual needs, setting realistic goals, designing balanced meal plans, and providing ongoing support, healthcare providers can empower expectant mothers to make informed dietary choices. This comprehensive approach not only promotes the health and development of the baby but also enhances the mother's overall wellbeing, contributing to a positive and healthy pregnancy journey.

As we conclude this comprehensive chapter on "Vital Vitamins, Mighty Minerals, and Supplements," it is evident that nutrition during pregnancy is a multifaceted journey requiring careful consideration and personalized attention. Throughout this chapter, we've explored the critical role that various vitamins and minerals play in supporting the health and development of both mother and baby. From the importance of folic acid in preventing neural tube defects to the role of iron in preventing anemia, each nutrient serves a unique and vital function during pregnancy.

We delved into the benefits, sources, and recommended dosages of essential vitamins such as Vitamin A, C, D, E, and the B-complex group. These vitamins are indispensable for maintaining maternal health, supporting fetal growth, and ensuring the smooth functioning of physiological processes. Similarly, we examined crucial minerals like calcium, iron, magnesium, and zinc, which are foundational for bone health, oxygen transport, enzymatic reactions, and immune function.

Understanding the role of supplements is equally important. Prenatal vitamins, omega-3 fatty acids, probiotics, vitamin D, iron, and calcium supplements can bridge nutritional gaps that diet alone may not cover. However, it is crucial to approach supplementation with care, considering potential interactions and the right dosages to avoid adverse effects.

This chapter also highlighted the significance of personalized nutrition planning, recognizing that every woman's pregnancy journey is unique. Tailoring nutrition plans to individual needs, preferences, and lifestyles ensures that both the mother and baby receive optimal nourishment. Through regular assessments, balanced meal plans, and professional guidance, personalized nutrition planning supports the overall wellbeing of the expectant mother.

In addition, we addressed the common challenges of morning sickness, cravings, and dietary aversions, offering practical solutions to maintain a balanced diet despite these hurdles. Recognizing and addressing nutrient deficiencies early on is critical to preventing complications and promoting a healthy pregnancy.

The journey of pregnancy is a transformative experience, and proper nutrition is the cornerstone of a healthy and joyful journey. Empowering expectant mothers with knowledge about vital vitamins, mighty minerals, and supplements allows them to make informed decisions that benefit their health and the development of their baby. By understanding the importance of these nutrients and how to incorporate them into their daily lives, mothers can confidently navigate their pregnancy with the assurance that they are providing the best possible foundation for their child's future.

In closing, remember that every pregnancy is unique, and while this chapter provides a general guide to prenatal nutrition, it is always essential to consult with healthcare providers for personalized advice. Embrace this journey with confidence, knowing that you have the tools and knowledge to nurture both yourself and your growing baby through optimal nutrition and wellness.

Chapter 4:

Hydration and Beverages

Welcome to Chapter 4 of The Nourished Pregnancy: A Self-Help Guide to Optimal Nutrition and Wellness. This chapter is designed to guide you through one of the most crucial aspects of pregnancy health – hydration and beverages. During pregnancy, not only does your body need more water to cope with the extra blood volume, but also to form amniotic fluid and support increased nutrient transport. Proper hydration is essential for maintaining your energy levels, supporting fetal development, and preventing common pregnancy complications such as constipation, urinary tract infections, and preterm labor.

In this chapter, we will explore various facets of hydration during pregnancy, starting with the fundamental importance of fluids and practical tips on how to ensure you're drinking enough. We'll dive into the specifics of caffeine consumption, its effects on you and your baby, and suggest healthier substitutes to keep you refreshed and energized. We'll then discuss the risks of alcohol consumption during pregnancy and provide alternative beverages that allow you to enjoy social events without compromising your health. Finally, we'll look into how maintaining adequate hydration can help prevent and manage pregnancy-related complications.

As you read through this chapter, remember that every sip you take contributes to the well-being of both you and your growing baby. Let's embark on this journey to better hydration and smarter beverage choices, ensuring a healthier and happier pregnancy.

Fluids for Two: Staying Hydrated

Staying hydrated is essential for everyone, but it is particularly crucial during pregnancy. When you're pregnant, your body's fluid needs increase significantly. Proper hydration supports the increased blood volume required to supply oxygen and nutrients to your baby. Additionally, water plays a vital role in forming amniotic fluid, aiding digestion, and helping to flush out waste and toxins.

Importance of Hydration during Pregnancy

Increased Blood Volume: As pregnancy progresses, your blood volume can increase by up to 50%. This extra blood helps deliver essential nutrients and oxygen to your baby and supports the increased metabolic demands of your body. Staying hydrated ensures that your blood volume is sufficient and that your circulation remains efficient.

Amniotic Fluid Production: Amniotic fluid surrounds and protects your baby in the womb. It acts as a cushion, provides room for growth and movement, and helps regulate your baby's temperature. Adequate hydration is essential for maintaining a healthy level of amniotic fluid.

Nutrient Transport: Water is a critical component of the body's transportation system. It helps carry nutrients from the food you eat to your baby and aids in the absorption of essential vitamins and minerals. Without adequate hydration, nutrient transport can be compromised, affecting your baby's growth and development.

Waste Removal: Your kidneys work harder during pregnancy to filter out waste products from both your body and your baby. Staying hydrated supports kidney function and helps prevent urinary tract infections (UTIs), which are more common during pregnancy.

Practical Tips for Staying Hydrated
Carry a Water Bottle: Keep a reusable water bottle with you at all times. Having water readily available makes it easier to sip throughout the day, ensuring you stay hydrated without having to make a conscious effort each time.

Set Reminders. Use your phone or a hydration app to set reminders to drink water regularly. This can be especially helpful if you get caught up in daily activities and forget to drink.

Flavor Your Water: If plain water isn't appealing, try adding natural flavors. Fresh fruit slices like lemon, lime, or cucumber can make water more enjoyable. Herbal teas, particularly those that are caffeine-free, can also be a good alternative.

Eat Hydrating Foods: Incorporate water-rich foods into your diet. Fruits like watermelon, strawberries, and oranges, and vegetables like cucumbers, lettuce, and celery have high water content and can contribute to your daily hydration needs.

Monitor Your Urine Color: A simple way to check your hydration status is by observing the color of your urine. Pale yellow indicates good hydration, while dark yellow or amber suggests you need to drink more fluids.

Drink Before You Feel Thirsty: Thirst is a sign that your body is already starting to become dehydrated. Make a habit of drinking water regularly throughout the day to prevent thirst from occurring.

Hydrate Before and After Exercise: If you're engaging in prenatal exercise, it's important to hydrate before, during, and after your workout to replace any fluids lost through sweat.

Limit Dehydrating Beverages: Reduce your intake of caffeinated and sugary drinks, as they can contribute to dehydration. Instead, opt for water, herbal teas, and natural fruit juices in moderation.

By following these tips, you can ensure that both you and your baby stay well-hydrated, promoting a healthier pregnancy and reducing the risk of complications.

Caffeine: How Much Is Too Much?

For many of us, a cup of coffee acts as a kick start to our day. However, during pregnancy, it's important to be aware of how much caffeine is safe. Caffeine is a stimulant that can cross the placenta and affect your baby's developing metabolism. Understanding the potential effects of caffeine and finding healthier substitutes can help you make informed choices for your and your baby's health.

Effects of Caffeine on Pregnancy
Increased Heart Rate and Blood Pressure: Caffeine can raise your heart rate and blood pressure. While moderate increases are generally safe, excessive caffeine intake can lead to significant spikes, which may affect your health and your baby's.

Diuretic Effects: Caffeine has diuretic properties, meaning it can increase urine production and potentially lead to dehydration. During pregnancy, staying hydrated is crucial, and excessive caffeine can counteract your hydration efforts.

Crossing the Placenta: Caffeine crosses the placenta, and because your baby's metabolism is still developing, they can't process caffeine as effectively as you can. This can lead to potential risks such as low birth weight or preterm birth.

Potential Miscarriage Risk: Some studies have suggested a link between high caffeine intake and an increased risk of miscarriage, particularly in the first trimester. While more research is needed, it's generally advised to limit caffeine intake to reduce potential risks.

Recommended Caffeine Limits

To minimize the risks associated with caffeine, health experts recommend limiting caffeine intake during pregnancy. The American College of Obstetricians and Gynecologists (ACOG) suggests that pregnant women should consume no more than 200 milligrams (mg) of caffeine per day. This is roughly equivalent to one 12-ounce cup of coffee.

Caffeine Content in Common Beverages and Foods

- ❖ Brewed Coffee (8 oz): 95-200 mg
- ❖ Black Tea (8 oz): 14-70 mg
- ❖ Green Tea (8 oz): 24-45 mg
- ❖ Cola (12 oz): 30-40 mg
- ❖ Energy Drinks (8 oz): 70-100 mg
- ❖ Dark Chocolate (1 oz): 12 mg
- ❖ Milk Chocolate (1 oz): 6 mg

Healthier Substitutes
Health authorities, including the American College of Obstetricians and Gynecologists (ACOG), recommend that pregnant women limit their caffeine intake to no more than 200 milligrams per day. This is roughly equivalent to one 12-ounce cup of coffee. It's important to remember that caffeine is also present in tea, chocolate, energy drinks, and some medications, so be mindful of all sources.

Healthier Substitutes for Caffeine
Herbal Teas: Herbal teas like chamomile, ginger, and peppermint can be soothing and provide a caffeine-free alternative to coffee and black tea. Always check with your healthcare provider before trying new herbal teas, as some herbs may not be safe during pregnancy.

Decaffeinated Coffee and Tea: If you love the taste of coffee or tea, consider switching to decaffeinated versions. These beverages have most of the caffeine removed but still offer the familiar flavors you enjoy.

Fruit-Infused Water: Create your own refreshing drinks by infusing water with slices of fruits like lemon, lime, orange, or berries. This can provide a natural boost of flavor without any caffeine.

Warm Milk: A glass of warm milk can be a comforting beverage that also provides essential nutrients like calcium and vitamin D. Add a touch of honey or a sprinkle of cinnamon for extra flavor.

Smoothies: Blend together your favorite fruits, yogurt, and a splash of milk or juice to create a nutritious and energizing smoothie. This can be a great way to start your day or enjoy as a mid-afternoon snack.

By being mindful of your caffeine intake and exploring these healthier alternatives, you can enjoy satisfying beverages without compromising your health or your baby's development.

Alcohol: The Risk and Alternatives

We understand that social situations can often revolve around alcohol, and it can be difficult feeling left out when you're pregnant. However, the risks posed by alcohol to prenatal development are significant. It's important to understand these risks and to find alternatives that allow you to enjoy social events without jeopardizing your health or that of your unborn child.

Risks of Alcohol Consumption During Pregnancy

Fetal Alcohol Spectrum Disorders (FASDs): Alcohol consumption during pregnancy can lead to a range of physical, behavioral, and cognitive issues known as Fetal Alcohol Spectrum Disorders. These disorders can include facial abnormalities, growth deficiencies, and central nervous system problems.

Developmental Delays: Exposure to alcohol in the womb can interfere with the normal development of the brain and other organs, leading to developmental delays and learning disabilities.

Low Birth Weight and Preterm Birth: Alcohol can restrict the growth of the fetus, resulting in low birth weight. It can also increase the risk of preterm birth, which can lead to additional health challenges for the newborn.

Miscarriage and Stillbirth: Drinking alcohol, especially in the first trimester, increases the risk of miscarriage and stillbirth.

Given these risks, no amount of alcohol is considered safe during pregnancy. The best approach is to abstain from alcohol entirely.

Sensible Alternatives to Alcohol
Mocktails: Enjoy non-alcoholic cocktails that are just as festive and flavorful as their alcoholic counterparts. Mix fresh fruit juices, sparkling water, and garnishes like mint or fruit slices to create delicious mocktails.

Non-Alcoholic Wine and Beer: Many brands offer non-alcoholic versions of wine and beer that mimic the taste and experience of traditional alcoholic beverages without the risks. These can be enjoyed in social settings to feel included.

Kombucha: While kombucha contains a small amount of alcohol due to fermentation, many pasteurized versions have minimal alcohol content and can be a refreshing alternative. Check with your healthcare provider to ensure it's safe for you.

Sparkling Water with a Twist: Jazz up your sparkling water with a splash of fruit juice or a squeeze of fresh citrus. This can provide a refreshing and festive drink that is perfect for social gatherings.

Herbal Teas and Infusions: Create a soothing and flavorful drink with herbal teas or infusions. Ingredients like hibiscus, chamomile, and ginger can make for a delightful beverage.

By choosing these alternatives, you can enjoy social events and celebrations without compromising your commitment to a healthy pregnancy.

Hydration and Pregnancy Complications

Dehydration during pregnancy isn't just about feeling thirsty or experiencing dry skin. It can lead to serious complications that affect both you and your baby. Proper hydration is crucial for preventing and managing these complications.

Common Pregnancy Complications Linked to Dehydration
Constipation: Dehydration can lead to constipation, which is a common issue during pregnancy due to hormonal changes and the pressure of the growing uterus on the intestines. Drinking enough water helps keep your digestive system functioning smoothly.

Urinary Tract Infections (UTIs): Pregnant women are more susceptible to UTIs, and dehydration can increase this risk. Staying well-hydrated helps flush bacteria from the urinary tract and can prevent infections.

Preterm Labor: Severe dehydration can trigger uterine contractions, potentially leading to preterm labor. Ensuring adequate hydration is essential for maintaining a healthy pregnancy duration.

Amniotic Fluid Levels: Adequate hydration helps maintain optimal levels of amniotic fluid, which is crucial for your baby's development and protection.

Swelling and Edema: While it may seem counterintuitive, drinking more water can help reduce swelling and edema. Proper hydration supports your body's natural balance and reduces fluid retention.

Headaches and Dizziness: Dehydration can cause headaches and dizziness, which can be particularly problematic during pregnancy. Staying hydrated helps prevent these uncomfortable symptoms.

Tips for Preventing Dehydration
Regular Fluid Intake: Make it a habit to drink water regularly throughout the day. Aim for at least 8-10 cups of water daily, and adjust based on your activity level and climate.

Hydrate with Meals: Drink a glass of water with each meal and snack. This not only helps with hydration but also aids in digestion.

Monitor Fluid Loss: Pay attention to how much you sweat, especially in hot weather or during exercise. Increase your fluid intake accordingly to compensate for any losses.

Avoid Diuretics: Limit beverages that have a diuretic effect, such as caffeinated drinks and sugary sodas. These can contribute to dehydration.

Listen to Your Body: Thirst is a natural signal that your body needs more fluids. Don't ignore it. Drink water as soon as you feel thirsty.

Infuse Variety: Make hydration enjoyable by varying your beverages. Incorporate herbal teas, flavored water, and water-rich foods to keep things interesting.

By maintaining proper hydration, you can help prevent these complications and ensure a smoother, healthier pregnancy.

In summary, hydration is a key component of a healthy pregnancy. By understanding the importance of fluids, making smart choices about caffeine and alcohol, and recognizing the role of hydration in preventing complications, you can support both your health and the health of your baby. Remember, every sip counts towards a nourished pregnancy.

Chapter 5:

Eating for Two: A Guide

Pregnancy is a unique and transformative period in a woman's life, marked by a series of physical, emotional, and nutritional changes. As you go on this remarkable journey, your body's nutritional needs will shift to support both your health and the optimal development of your baby. "Eating for Two: A Guide" is designed to help you navigate these changes with confidence and ease. This chapter will provide you with a comprehensive understanding of the essential nutrients required during pregnancy, practical tips for maintaining a balanced diet, and delicious, nutritious meal ideas that cater to your unique needs.

We'll start by exploring the Pregnancy Food Pyramid, a tailored version of the traditional food pyramid that emphasizes the importance of specific food groups and their roles in pregnancy. You'll learn about the significance of grains, proteins, healthy fats, fruits and vegetables, and dairy and calcium, along with practical ways to incorporate these foods into your daily diet.

Next, we'll address the challenges of maintaining a healthy diet on the go. Life doesn't pause for pregnancy, and whether you're juggling work, family, or other responsibilities, it's crucial to have strategies for healthy snacking, meal planning, and eating out. We'll provide you with tips on how to make nutritious choices even when you're busy or dining away from home.

Managing cravings and aversions is another key aspect of pregnancy nutrition. We'll delve into the reasons behind these changes in taste and appetite, offering healthy ways to satisfy your cravings and manage aversions without compromising your nutritional intake.

We'll also introduce you to a variety of pregnancy-friendly foods and recipes. These meal ideas are not only nutritious but also designed to be satisfying and enjoyable, helping you meet your dietary needs while indulging in delicious flavors.

Finally, we'll provide a detailed 7-day meal plan along with a comprehensive grocery list. This practical guide will help you apply the nutritional advice from this chapter in your everyday life, ensuring that you and your baby receive the essential nutrients needed for a healthy and thriving pregnancy.

So, let's embark on this nourishing journey together. Whether you're a first-time mom or adding another member to your family, this chapter will equip you with the knowledge and confidence to eat well and feel great throughout your pregnancy.

The Pregnancy Food Pyramid

Whole grains form the foundation of a healthy pregnancy diet. These nutrient-dense foods are a primary source of energy, providing complex carbohydrates, fiber, vitamins, and minerals essential for both mother and baby. During pregnancy, it's important to focus on whole grains rather than refined grains to maximize nutritional benefits.

Carbohydrates are the body's main source of energy. Whole grains, such as oats, brown rice, quinoa, and whole wheat, provide sustained energy due to their complex carbohydrate content. This helps to combat fatigue, a common symptom during pregnancy.

Whole grains are rich in dietary fiber, which aids digestion and helps prevent constipation, a common issue for pregnant women. Fiber also helps regulate blood sugar levels, reducing the risk of gestational diabetes.

Whole grains are packed with essential nutrients such as B vitamins (including folic acid), iron, magnesium, and selenium. Folic acid is particularly crucial in the early stages of pregnancy for preventing neural tube defects in the developing fetus.

Pregnant women should aim to consume 6-8 servings of grains per day, with at least half of these servings coming from whole grains. One serving of grains can be equivalent to:

- ✓ 1 slice of whole-grain bread
- ✓ 1/2 cup of cooked brown rice or quinoa
- ✓ 1/2 cup of whole-grain pasta
- ✓ 1 cup of ready-to-eat whole-grain cereal
- ✓ 1/2 cup of cooked oatmeal

Start your day with a hearty bowl of oatmeal topped with fresh fruit and a sprinkle of nuts or seeds. Whole-grain cereals or whole-wheat toast with avocado are also excellent choices.

Incorporate whole grains into your lunch with a quinoa salad mixed with vegetables, chickpeas, and a light dressing. Alternatively, a sandwich made with whole-grain bread, lean protein, and plenty of veggies is a balanced option.

Use brown rice or whole-grain pasta as a base for your evening meals. Pair with lean proteins and a variety of vegetables to create a nutritious and satisfying dish.

Whole-grain crackers with hummus or a slice of whole-grain bread with nut butter can make for a healthy and filling snack.

When baking at home, opt for whole-grain flour instead of refined white flour. This simple switch can significantly boost the nutritional value of your baked goods.

Protein is a critical component of a healthy pregnancy diet, playing a vital role in the growth and development of the baby as well as the health of the mother. During pregnancy, the body's protein requirements increase to support the formation of fetal tissues, including the brain, muscles, and other vital organs.

Protein is the building block of cells and is essential for the growth and repair of tissues. Adequate protein intake supports the development of your baby's organs, muscles, and brain.

Protein helps maintain maternal tissues, supports increased blood volume, and aids in the production of hormones and enzymes. It also contributes to a healthy immune system, helping to protect both mother and baby from infections.

Protein can help manage weight gain during pregnancy by promoting a feeling of fullness and reducing the likelihood of overeating.

Pregnant women should aim to consume about 70-100 grams of protein per day. This can vary based on individual needs and body weight. High-quality protein sources include:

- ✓ Lean meats (chicken, turkey, beef, pork)
- ✓ Fish (low-mercury options like salmon, trout, and sardines)
- ✓ Eggs

✓ Dairy products (milk, cheese, yogurt)
✓ Legumes (beans, lentils, chickpeas)
✓ Nuts and seeds
✓ Soy products (tofu, tempeh, edamame)

Start your day with protein-rich options like eggs, Greek yogurt with nuts and fruit, or a smoothie made with protein powder, spinach, and almond milk.

Include lean proteins in your lunch, such as a grilled chicken salad, a turkey and avocado sandwich on whole-grain bread, or a lentil and vegetable soup.

Opt for protein-packed dinners like baked salmon with quinoa and steamed vegetables, stir-fried tofu with brown rice and mixed veggies, or a beef and vegetable stew.

Healthy snacks can include a handful of nuts, a hard-boiled egg, cottage cheese with fruit, or hummus with veggie sticks.

Ensure you're getting a variety of protein sources to cover a broad spectrum of nutrients. For example, include both animal and plant-based proteins in your diet.

Fats are a necessary part of a balanced diet, especially during pregnancy. They provide energy, support the absorption of fat-soluble vitamins, and are essential for the development of the baby's brain and eyes.

Essential fatty acids, particularly omega-3 fatty acids (DHA and EPA), are crucial for the development of the fetal brain and retina. These fats are important for cognitive and visual development.

Fats are a concentrated source of energy. During pregnancy, your caloric needs increase, and healthy fats can help meet these additional energy requirements.

Fats help in the absorption of fat-soluble vitamins such as vitamins A, D, E, and K. These vitamins are vital for both maternal and fetal health.

While the exact amount of fat needed can vary, it is generally recommended that about 20-35% of your daily calories come from fat, with a focus on healthy fats. Good sources of healthy fats include:

✓ Avocados
✓ Nuts and seeds (almonds, walnuts, chia seeds, flaxseeds)
✓ Olive oil and other vegetable oils
✓ Fatty fish (salmon, mackerel, sardines)
✓ Nut butters
✓ Dark chocolate (in moderation)

Add avocado slices to your whole-grain toast, sprinkle chia seeds or flaxseeds on your oatmeal, or include nuts in your morning yogurt.

Use olive oil-based dressings for salads, include nuts and seeds in your meals, or enjoy a serving of fatty fish like salmon in your sandwich or salad.

Cook with healthy oils such as olive oil or canola oil. Include dishes like grilled fish with a side of vegetables, or a stir-fry with tofu and sesame oil.

Enjoy a handful of nuts, a piece of dark chocolate, or veggie sticks with guacamole. Nut butters on apple slices or whole-grain crackers can also be a satisfying snack.

Use healthy fats in your cooking and baking. Replace butter with olive oil or avocado oil, and incorporate more fatty fish into your meals.

Fruits and vegetables are vital components of a healthy pregnancy diet, providing essential vitamins, minerals, fiber, and antioxidants that support both maternal and fetal health.

Fruits and vegetables are packed with vitamins and minerals, including vitamin C, vitamin A, folate, potassium, and fiber. These nutrients are crucial for the health of the mother and the developing baby.

Many fruits and vegetables have high water content, helping to maintain hydration, which is important for overall health and preventing common pregnancy issues like constipation.

The antioxidants in fruits and vegetables help protect the body from oxidative stress and inflammation, promoting a healthy immune system.

Pregnant women should aim to consume at least 5 servings of fruits and vegetables per day, with a focus on variety and color to ensure a broad range of nutrients. Examples of one serving include:

- ✓ 1 medium-sized fruit (apple, banana, orange)
- ✓ 1/2 cup of fresh, frozen, or canned fruit (in 100% juice)
- ✓ 1 cup of raw leafy vegetables (spinach, kale, lettuce)
- ✓ 1/2 cup of cooked vegetables (broccoli, carrots, bell peppers)
- ✓ 1/2 cup of 100% fruit or vegetable juice

Start your day with a fruit smoothie, a bowl of mixed berries, or add vegetables like spinach and tomatoes to your omelet.

Include a variety of vegetables in your salads, add slices of cucumber, bell pepper, and tomato to your sandwiches, or enjoy a bowl of vegetable soup.

Serve a side of steamed or roasted vegetables with your main course, make a vegetable stir-fry, or incorporate veggies into your pasta dishes.

Keep fresh fruits like apples, bananas, and grapes on hand for easy snacks. Enjoy raw vegetable sticks with hummus or yogurt dip.

Experiment with different cooking methods to keep things interesting. Try grilling, steaming, roasting, or sautéing vegetables to bring out their flavors.

Dairy products are an important part of a balanced diet during pregnancy, providing essential nutrients such as calcium, protein, vitamin D, and phosphorus, which are vital for the development of the baby's bones and teeth.

Calcium is crucial for the development of the baby's bones and teeth. It also helps maintain the mother's bone density, preventing the body from depleting maternal calcium stores.

Calcium plays a role in muscle contractions and nerve transmission, helping to prevent muscle cramps and support overall muscle function.

Dairy products contain vitamin D, which is essential for calcium absorption and plays a role in regulating hormones that support pregnancy.

Pregnant women should aim for about 1,000 mg of calcium per day, which can be met through 3-4 servings of dairy or other calcium-rich foods. Good sources of calcium include:

- ✓ Milk (cow's milk, fortified plant-based milks)
- ✓ Cheese (cheddar, mozzarella, cottage cheese)
- ✓ Yogurt (Greek yogurt, regular yogurt)
- ✓ Leafy green vegetables (kale, broccoli)
- ✓ Fortified foods (orange juice, cereals)
- ✓ Tofu and tempeh
- ✓ Almonds and sesame seeds

Enjoy a bowl of fortified cereal with milk, Greek yogurt with fresh fruit, or a smoothie made with fortified plant-based milk.

Include cheese in your sandwiches or salads, have a serving of cottage cheese with fruit, or enjoy a cup of milk with your meal.

Incorporate dairy into your dinner by adding cheese to your pasta dishes, making creamy soups with milk, or having a side of yogurt with your meal.

Snack on cheese sticks, yogurt, or a glass of milk. Fortified plant-based milks and calcium-fortified orange juice are also excellent options.

Use dairy products in your cooking and baking. Add milk or cheese to your casseroles, make smoothies with yogurt, or use fortified plant-based milk in your recipes.

By following the Pregnancy Food Pyramid and incorporating a variety of grains, proteins, healthy fats, fruits and vegetables, and dairy into your diet, you can ensure that you and your baby receive the essential nutrients needed for a healthy and thriving pregnancy.

<u>Eating on the Go: Healthy Options</u>

Life doesn't stop when you're pregnant, and there will be days when you're on the go. Maintaining a healthy diet during these times is crucial for keeping your energy levels up and ensuring you and your baby get the nutrients you need. Healthy snacking can be a lifesaver in these situations.

Regular snacking can prevent extreme hunger that leads to overeating during main meals. It also helps stabilize blood sugar levels, reducing the risk of gestational diabetes.

Maintaining a healthy diet while on the go can be challenging, especially during pregnancy when your nutritional needs are heightened. This section will provide practical advice on how to keep up with your healthy eating habits even when life gets busy. We'll cover healthy snacking, meal planning and grocery shopping tips, eating out and ordering in, and meal prep and batch cooking for pregnancy.

Healthy Snacking

Snacking can be a crucial part of a pregnant woman's diet, helping to keep energy levels stable and prevent excessive hunger that can lead to overeating at meal times. Here are some healthy snacking tips:

Benefits of Healthy Snacking

Maintains Energy Levels: Frequent, small snacks can help sustain your energy throughout the day, preventing fatigue and keeping you alert.

Meets Nutritional Needs: Healthy snacks can help you meet your daily nutritional requirements, especially if your main meals are sometimes rushed or lacking in certain nutrients.

Prevents Overeating: Regular snacking can prevent extreme hunger that leads to overeating during main meals. It also helps stabilize blood sugar levels, reducing the risk of gestational diabetes.

Healthy Snack Ideas

Fruits and Vegetables: Fresh fruits like apples, bananas, and berries are portable and nutritious. Vegetables like carrot sticks, celery, and cherry tomatoes can be paired with hummus or yogurt dip for added flavor.

Nuts and Seeds: A handful of almonds, walnuts, or sunflower seeds can provide healthy fats, protein, and fiber.

Dairy Products: Yogurt, cheese sticks, and smoothies made with milk or fortified plant-based milk are excellent options. Greek yogurt with a drizzle of honey and a sprinkle of nuts is both satisfying and nutritious.

Whole Grains: Whole grain crackers, rice cakes, and granola bars can offer sustained energy. Look for options low in added sugars and high in fiber.

Protein-Rich Snacks: Hard-boiled eggs, edamame, and chickpeas are convenient sources of protein. Consider making a batch of protein balls using oats, nut butter, and seeds.

Meal Planning and Grocery Shopping Tips

Effective meal planning and smart grocery shopping can help you maintain a balanced diet without much hassle. Here are some strategies to consider:

Meal Planning

Plan Ahead: Take some time each week to plan your meals and snacks. This helps ensure you have all the ingredients you need and reduces the likelihood of resorting to unhealthy options.

Balanced Meals: Ensure each meal includes a balance of carbohydrates, proteins, and fats. This will help you stay full and energized throughout the day.

Prepare for Cravings: Plan for healthier alternatives to common pregnancy cravings. For example, if you crave sweets, have some fruit or yogurt on hand instead of candy.

Batch Cooking: Prepare larger quantities of meals that can be stored and eaten throughout the week. This saves time and ensures you always have something healthy to eat.

Grocery Shopping Tips

Make a List: Always shop with a list based on your meal plan. This helps you avoid impulse buys and ensures you get everything you need.

Shop the Perimeter: Most grocery stores have fresh produce, dairy, and meats around the perimeter of the store. Focus on these areas to find healthier options.

Read Labels: Check food labels for added sugars, unhealthy fats, and excessive sodium. Opt for whole foods with minimal processing.

Buy in Bulk: Items like grains, nuts, and seeds can be bought in bulk, saving money and ensuring you always have healthy ingredients on hand.

Seasonal Produce: Choose fruits and vegetables that are in season. They are usually fresher, more nutritious, and more affordable.

Eating Out and Ordering In

Eating out or ordering in doesn't have to derail your healthy eating habits. Here are some tips to make better choices:

Eating Out

Choose Wisely: Look for restaurants that offer healthy options. Many places now provide nutritional information on their menus.

Portion Control: Restaurant portions are often larger than what you need. Consider sharing a dish or asking for a half portion.

Customize Your Order: Don't hesitate to ask for modifications. Request dressings and sauces on the side, opt for grilled instead of fried items, and add extra vegetables to your meal.

Healthy Starters: Start with a salad or a broth-based soup to fill up on low-calorie, nutrient-dense foods.

Drink Smart: Choose water, sparkling water, or unsweetened tea instead of sugary drinks or alcohol.

Ordering In

Choose Healthier Cuisines: Opt for cuisines that offer balanced meals with lots of vegetables, lean proteins, and whole grains. Mediterranean, Japanese, and Thai are often good choices.

Be Mindful of Extras: Skip the sides like fries or breadsticks and avoid sugary desserts.

Include a Salad: Order a side salad to add more vegetables to your meal.

Watch Portions: Just like eating out, be mindful of portions when ordering in. Save half for another meal if the portion is too large.

Meal Prep and Batch Cooking for Pregnancy

Preparing meals in advance can be a game-changer, especially when you're juggling a busy schedule and pregnancy. Here are some tips for effective meal prep and batch cooking:

Benefits of Meal Prep

Saves Time: Prepping meals ahead of time means you spend less time cooking during the week.

Reduces Stress: Having meals ready to go reduces the stress of figuring out what to eat, especially on busy days.

Ensures Balanced Meals: Pre-planned meals help ensure you're getting a balanced diet without resorting to unhealthy options.

Meal Prep Tips

Start Simple: Begin with easy-to-make meals that can be prepared in large quantities. Soups, stews, casseroles, and grain bowls are great options.

Use Storage Containers: Invest in good-quality storage containers that can be easily stacked in your refrigerator or freezer.

Label Everything: Clearly label containers with the date and contents to keep track of what needs to be eaten first.

Prep Ingredients: Wash and chop vegetables, cook grains and proteins, and portion out snacks so they're ready to grab and go.

Batch Cooking Ideas

Soups and Stews: Make a big pot of soup or stew that can be frozen in individual portions. These are nutrient-dense and easy to reheat.

Grain Bowls: Cook a large batch of quinoa, brown rice, or farro. Combine with roasted vegetables, beans, and a protein source for quick and nutritious meals.

Breakfast Options: Prepare overnight oats, smoothie packs, or egg muffins for easy breakfasts.

Healthy Snacks: Make batches of energy balls, granola bars, or trail mix to have healthy snacks on hand.

By incorporating these strategies into your routine, you can maintain a healthy diet even when life gets busy. Healthy snacking, effective meal planning, smart choices when eating out, and batch cooking will help you stay on track and ensure you and your baby get the nutrition you need.

Managing Cravings and Aversions

Pregnancy often brings about significant changes in appetite and taste preferences. Understanding and managing cravings and aversions is essential to maintaining a balanced diet. This section will help you navigate these changes, offering insights into why they occur and how to handle them healthily.

Understanding Cravings and Aversions
Cravings and aversions during pregnancy are common, often driven by hormonal changes. Here's a deeper look into these phenomena:

Hormonal Influences: Hormonal fluctuations, particularly increased levels of estrogen and progesterone, can alter taste and smell, making certain foods more appealing or repulsive.

Nutritional Needs: Sometimes, cravings might indicate a nutritional deficiency. For example, craving red meat could signal a need for more iron, while a desire for dairy might reflect a need for calcium.

Emotional Factors: Pregnancy can be a stressful time, and cravings can sometimes be linked to emotional comfort. Comfort foods often have a nostalgic or soothing effect, helping to alleviate stress.

Common Cravings and Aversions: Cravings vary widely but often include sweet, salty, or spicy foods. Conversely, aversions typically involve strong-tasting or -smelling foods, such as garlic, onions, or certain meats.

Healthy Ways to Satisfy Cravings
While it's okay to indulge occasionally, it's important to satisfy cravings in a healthy manner to ensure you and your baby are getting the necessary nutrients. Here are some strategies:

Balance is Key: If you're craving something sweet, opt for a piece of fruit or yogurt with honey. For salty cravings, try air-popped popcorn with a sprinkle of sea salt instead of chips.

Portion Control: If you must have your favorite indulgence, practice portion control. A small piece of dark chocolate can satisfy a sweet tooth without overindulgence.

Healthy Alternatives: Look for healthier versions of your cravings. For example, if you crave ice cream, try a homemade smoothie with frozen bananas and a splash of milk. Craving something crunchy? Opt for raw veggies with hummus.

Mindful Eating: Pay attention to why you're craving certain foods. Sometimes, drinking a glass of water or going for a walk can reduce cravings.

Nutrient-Dense Foods: Incorporate nutrient-dense foods into your diet to help curb cravings. Foods rich in protein, fiber, and healthy fats can help you feel fuller for longer, reducing the likelihood of unhealthy snacking.

Managing Aversions and Food Avoidances
Dealing with food aversions can be tricky, especially when those foods are important for your nutrition. Here are some tips to manage aversions while still meeting your dietary needs:

Find Alternatives: If you can't stand the thought of a particular food, find alternatives that provide similar nutrients. For example, if you're averse to meat, try plant-based protein sources like beans, lentils, or tofu.

Modify Preparation: Sometimes, changing how a food is prepared can make it more palatable. If the smell of cooked fish is off-putting, try consuming it cold in a salad or sandwich.

Incorporate Small Amounts: Gradually reintroduce small amounts of the averted food into your diet. Mixing it with other foods can help mask the taste and make it more tolerable.

Nutrient Supplements: If aversions are preventing you from getting essential nutrients, talk to your healthcare provider about supplements. They can recommend safe and effective options to ensure you're meeting your nutritional needs.

Stay Hydrated: Sometimes, aversions can be exacerbated by dehydration. Drinking plenty of water throughout the day can help reduce the intensity of aversions.

Additional Tips

Listen to Your Body: Pay attention to what your body is telling you. Cravings and aversions can be signals of what your body needs or doesn't need at the moment.

Stay Flexible: It's important to be flexible with your diet during pregnancy. If you find that you can't stick to your usual eating habits, don't stress. Focus on making the best choices you can each day.

Seek Support: If you're struggling with extreme cravings or aversions, seek support from a nutritionist or healthcare provider. They can offer personalized advice and reassurance.

Keep a Food Diary: Keeping track of what you eat and how you feel can help identify patterns and triggers for cravings and aversions. This can be useful information for discussing with your healthcare provider.

By understanding and managing cravings and aversions, you can maintain a balanced diet that supports both your health and your baby's development. The key is to find healthy ways to satisfy your cravings and find alternatives or modifications for foods you can't tolerate.

Pregnancy-Friendly Foods and Recipes

Eating nutritious foods during pregnancy is essential for the health of both mother and baby. However, it can sometimes be challenging to find meals that are both healthy and satisfying, especially when dealing with pregnancy cravings and aversions. This section provides a range of nutritious and delicious meal ideas, healthier twists on comfort foods, and recipes for common pregnancy cravings.

Nutritious and Delicious Meal Ideas

Breakfast:

Overnight Oats: Combine oats with milk or a dairy-free alternative, chia seeds, and your favorite fruits. Let it sit overnight, and in the morning, top with nuts and a drizzle of honey. This meal is packed with fiber, protein, and essential vitamins.

Greek Yogurt Parfait: Layer Greek yogurt with granola, fresh berries, and a sprinkle of flaxseeds. Greek yogurt provides a good source of protein and probiotics, which are beneficial for gut health.

Avocado Toast: Spread mashed avocado on whole-grain toast and top with a poached egg. Avocado is rich in healthy fats, and eggs provide protein and choline, which is important for fetal brain development.

Lunch:
 Quinoa Salad: Mix cooked quinoa with chopped vegetables like bell peppers, cucumbers, and tomatoes. Add in some chickpeas or grilled chicken for protein, and dress with olive oil and lemon juice. Quinoa is a complete protein and provides essential amino acids.
Vegetable Soup: Prepare a hearty vegetable soup with carrots, celery, tomatoes, spinach, and beans. This soup is rich in vitamins, minerals, and fiber, making it a nutritious and filling option.
Chicken Wrap: Use a whole-grain tortilla and fill it with grilled chicken, mixed greens, avocado, and a light vinaigrette. This wrap provides a balanced mix of protein, healthy fats, and fiber.

Dinner:
 Baked Salmon with Sweet Potato: Season salmon with lemon, garlic, and herbs, then bake alongside sweet potato wedges. Salmon is high in omega-3 fatty acids, which are crucial for fetal brain development.
Stir-Fried Tofu with Vegetables: Stir-fry tofu with broccoli, bell peppers, snap peas, and a soy-ginger sauce. Tofu is an excellent plant-based protein source, and the vegetables provide a variety of essential nutrients.
Spaghetti Squash with Marinara Sauce: Roast spaghetti squash and top with homemade marinara sauce and a sprinkle of parmesan cheese. Spaghetti squash is a low-calorie, nutrient-dense alternative to traditional pasta.

Healthy Twists on Comfort Foods
Cauliflower Pizza: Use a cauliflower crust instead of traditional dough and top with tomato sauce, cheese, and your favorite vegetables. This version is lower in carbs and higher in fiber.
Zucchini Noodles: Swap out pasta for spiraled zucchini noodles, also known as zoodles. Serve with a pesto sauce or marinara for a lighter, nutrient-packed meal.
Baked Sweet Potato Fries: Instead of regular fries, opt for baked sweet potato fries. They are rich in beta-carotene and other vitamins, making them a healthier alternative.
Greek Yogurt Ice Cream: Blend Greek yogurt with frozen berries and a bit of honey for a delicious and protein-rich ice cream alternative.
Black Bean Brownies: Substitute some or all of the flour in your brownie recipe with black beans. This adds fiber and protein while keeping the dessert indulgent and satisfying.

Recipes for Common Pregnancy Cravings

Sweet Cravings:
Fruit Smoothies: Blend together a banana, a handful of spinach, a cup of frozen berries, and some almond milk. This smoothie is sweet, satisfying, and packed with nutrients.
Dark Chocolate-Covered Strawberries: Dip fresh strawberries in melted dark chocolate. Dark chocolate has less sugar than milk chocolate and provides antioxidants.

Salty Cravings:
Kale Chips: Toss kale leaves with olive oil and a sprinkle of sea salt, then bake until crispy. Kale chips are a crunchy, salty snack that's rich in vitamins A, C, and K.
Roasted Chickpeas: Season chickpeas with your favorite spices and roast until crispy. They make a great snack that's high in protein and fiber.

Spicy Cravings:
Stuffed Bell Peppers: Fill bell peppers with a mixture of quinoa, black beans, corn, and a spicy tomato sauce. Bake until the peppers are tender.
Spicy Hummus: Blend chickpeas with tahini, lemon juice, garlic, and a dash of cayenne pepper. Serve with fresh vegetables or whole-grain pita chips.
Additional Tips
Meal Prepping: Prepare larger batches of meals and freeze them in individual portions. This can make it easier to stick to a healthy diet, even on busy days.
Stay Hydrated: Drink plenty of water throughout the day, and include hydrating foods like cucumbers, watermelon, and oranges in your diet.
Listen to Your Body: Pay attention to your hunger and fullness cues. Eating small, frequent meals can help manage hunger and prevent overeating.

By incorporating these nutritious and delicious meal ideas, healthier comfort food alternatives, and satisfying recipes for common cravings, you can enjoy a balanced and enjoyable diet throughout your pregnancy.
 Throughout this chapter, we have explored the art and science of eating for two during pregnancy, focusing on essential aspects such as the Pregnancy Food Pyramid, eating healthy on the go, managing cravings and aversions, and preparing pregnancy-friendly foods and recipes.

Key Takeaways:

❖ The Pregnancy Food Pyramid: Understanding the importance of grains, protein, healthy fats, fruits and vegetables, and dairy and calcium in your diet during pregnancy ensures you're meeting both your needs and your baby's developmental requirements.

❖ Eating on the Go: Practical tips for healthy snacking, meal planning, grocery shopping, eating out, and meal prep have equipped you with strategies to maintain a nutritious diet despite a busy lifestyle.

❖ Managing Cravings and Aversions: Recognizing the hormonal, nutritional, and emotional factors behind cravings and aversions has empowered you to make informed choices and find healthier alternatives to satisfy your palate.

❖ Pregnancy-Friendly Foods and Recipes: From nutritious meal ideas to healthier twists on comfort foods and recipes for common cravings, you now have a repertoire of delicious options to enjoy while supporting your baby's growth and development.

As you continue your pregnancy journey, remember to listen to your body, stay hydrated, and seek support from healthcare professionals for personalized guidance. Every meal you enjoy is an opportunity to nourish yourself and your baby with the nutrients essential for a healthy pregnancy.

Chapter 6:

Active and Healthy

Welcome to Chapter 6 of "The Nourished Pregnancy: A Self-Help Guide to Optimal Nutrition and Wellness." In this chapter, titled "Active and Healthy," we explore the critical role of physical activity in ensuring a healthy and enjoyable pregnancy. Staying active during pregnancy offers numerous benefits, from boosting mood and energy levels to alleviating common discomforts such as back pain and swelling. Regular exercise can also enhance sleep, reduce stress, and prepare your body for the demands of labor and delivery.

Pregnancy is a time of significant physical and emotional changes. Understanding how to maintain an active lifestyle safely and effectively can make a substantial difference in your overall well-being. This chapter will guide you through various aspects of exercising during pregnancy, providing practical tips, safety guidelines, and motivational advice.

We'll begin by discussing the benefits of physical activity during pregnancy, along with essential tips and precautions to keep in mind. From there, we'll explore how to modify your exercise routine to accommodate the unique needs of your changing body, including specific exercises like pelvic floor workouts and stretching. Next, we'll delve into trimester-specific exercise guidelines, helping you adapt your activities as your pregnancy progresses. Finally, we'll offer advice on getting started with an exercise routine, staying motivated, and overcoming common barriers.

By the end of this chapter, you'll have a comprehensive understanding of how to stay active and healthy throughout your pregnancy, empowering you to make informed decisions that benefit both you and your baby. Let's embark on this journey towards a fit and healthy pregnancy together!

Active and Healthy Physical Activity: Tips and Precautions

The role of exercise in a healthy pregnancy cannot be overstated. Engaging in regular physical activity offers numerous benefits for both the expectant mother and the developing baby.

Exercise helps alleviate common pregnancy symptoms such as fatigue, constipation, and morning sickness, and it plays a vital role in preparing your body for labor and delivery. Additionally, staying active can help manage weight gain, reduce the risk of gestational diabetes, and improve mental health by reducing stress and anxiety.

Benefits of Exercise During Pregnancy:

- ❖ Improved Mood and Energy Levels: Regular physical activity can boost your mood and energy levels by releasing endorphins, the body's natural feel-good hormones. This can help combat the emotional ups and downs that often accompany pregnancy.
- ❖ Better Sleep: Exercise can promote better sleep by helping you fall asleep faster and enjoy deeper, more restful sleep. This is particularly beneficial during pregnancy when sleep can be disrupted by physical discomfort and hormonal changes.
- ❖ Reduced Pregnancy Discomforts: Physical activity can alleviate common pregnancy discomforts such as back pain, swelling, and constipation. Strengthening muscles and improving circulation can reduce the aches and pains associated with pregnancy.
- ❖ Preparation for Labor and Delivery: Staying active helps build stamina and strength, which are essential for labor and delivery. Exercises that strengthen the pelvic floor muscles, such as Kegels, can also facilitate a smoother delivery and quicker postpartum recovery.
- ❖ Lower Risk of Gestational Diabetes: Regular exercise can help regulate blood sugar levels, reducing the risk of gestational diabetes. This is important for the health of both the mother and the baby.
- ❖ Weight Management: Exercise helps manage healthy weight gain during pregnancy, reducing the risk of excessive weight gain and associated complications.

Safety Guidelines and Precautions:
While the benefits of exercise during pregnancy are numerous, it's crucial to follow safety guidelines to protect both you and your baby. Here are some essential precautions to keep in mind:

1. Consult Your Healthcare Provider: Before starting any exercise routine, consult your healthcare provider to ensure that it's safe for you and your baby. This is especially important if you have any pre-existing medical conditions or pregnancy complications.
2. Stay Hydrated: Drink plenty of water before, during, and after exercise to stay hydrated. Dehydration can lead to overheating and other complications.

3. Avoid Overheating: Exercise in a cool environment and avoid activities that can cause overheating, such as hot yoga. Overheating can be harmful to both you and your baby.

4. Wear Comfortable Clothing and Supportive Shoes: Choose loose, comfortable clothing and wear supportive shoes to reduce the risk of injury and discomfort.

5. Listen to Your Body: Pay attention to your body's signals and adjust your exercise routine as needed. If you experience any pain, dizziness, shortness of breath, or unusual symptoms, stop exercising and consult your healthcare provider.

6. Avoid High-Impact Activities: Avoid high-impact activities and contact sports that carry a risk of injury or falling. Instead, focus on low-impact exercises that are safe and gentle on your body.

Types of Exercises Suitable for Pregnancy:

1. Prenatal Yoga: Prenatal yoga is an excellent form of exercise for pregnant women. It helps improve flexibility, strength, and balance while promoting relaxation and stress relief. Prenatal yoga poses are designed to accommodate the changes in your body and provide relief from common pregnancy discomforts.

2. Swimming: Swimming is a low-impact exercise that provides a full-body workout. The buoyancy of the water supports your weight, reducing strain on your joints and muscles. Swimming can also help alleviate swelling and improve circulation.

3. Walking: Walking is a simple and effective way to stay active during pregnancy. It's low-impact and can be easily incorporated into your daily routine. Aim for at least 30 minutes of walking most days of the week to reap the benefits.

By following these tips and precautions, you can enjoy the benefits of physical activity while ensuring the safety and well-being of both you and your baby.

Special Considerations: Modifying Your Routine

Just as every pregnancy is unique, so should be every exercise routine. Listening to your body and making necessary adjustments based on its responses is crucial for a healthy and safe pregnancy. This section will guide you on how to modify your exercise routine to accommodate your changing body and ensure you stay active without compromising safety.

Adjusting Exercise Intensity and Frequency:

1. Listen to Your Body: Pregnancy is not the time to push your limits. Pay attention to your body's signals and adjust the intensity and frequency of your workouts accordingly. If you feel fatigued or experience any discomfort, take a break or reduce the intensity of your exercise.
2. Modify Your Workouts: As your pregnancy progresses, certain exercises may become more challenging or uncomfortable. Modify your workouts to match your energy levels and physical capabilities. For example, if running becomes too strenuous, switch to brisk walking or swimming.
3. Pace Yourself: Maintain a moderate pace that allows you to talk comfortably without becoming breathless. The "talk test" is a good indicator of whether you're exercising at an appropriate intensity.

Avoiding High-Impact Activities and Contact Sports:

1. High-Impact Activities: Avoid high-impact activities such as running, jumping, and aerobics that can put excessive strain on your joints and increase the risk of injury. Instead, opt for low-impact exercises like walking, swimming, and stationary cycling.
2. Contact Sports: Steer clear of contact sports like basketball, soccer, and martial arts, as they carry a higher risk of injury and impact. These activities can lead to falls, collisions, and abdominal trauma, which can be harmful to you and your baby.
3. Activities with a Risk of Falling: Avoid activities that carry a risk of falling, such as skiing, horseback riding, and mountain biking. Falls can pose a serious risk to both you and your baby.

Incorporating Pelvic Floor Exercises (Kegels) and Stretching:

1. Pelvic Floor Exercises (Kegels): Strengthening your pelvic floor muscles is essential during pregnancy. Kegel exercises involve contracting and relaxing the pelvic floor muscles, which support the uterus, bladder, and bowels. These exercises can help prevent urinary incontinence, reduce the risk of pelvic organ prolapse, and improve your ability to push during labor.
   - How to Perform Kegels: To perform Kegel exercises, tighten your pelvic floor muscles as if you're trying to stop the flow of urine. Hold the contraction for a few seconds, then release. Repeat this exercise 10-15 times, several times a day.
2. Stretching: Gentle stretching can help improve flexibility, reduce muscle tension, and alleviate pregnancy-related discomforts such as back pain and tightness. Incorporate stretching into your daily routine, focusing on areas like the lower back, hips, and legs.
   - Safe Stretching Tips: Avoid overstretching and bouncing during stretches. Hold each stretch for 15-30 seconds and breathe deeply. Stretching should feel gentle and comfortable, not painful.

Creating a Safe and Effective Exercise Routine:

1. Warm-Up and Cool-Down: Always begin your exercise routine with a warm-up to prepare your muscles and joints for activity. A proper warm-up increases blood flow and reduces the risk of injury. Similarly, end your workout with a cool-down to gradually lower your heart rate and stretch your muscles.
2. Balanced Routine: Incorporate a variety of exercises into your routine, including cardiovascular, strength, and flexibility exercises. This balanced approach ensures you target different muscle groups and maintain overall fitness.
3. Stay Hydrated and Nourished: Drink plenty of water before, during, and after exercise to stay hydrated. Additionally, fuel your body with nutritious foods to support your energy levels and overall health.

By modifying your exercise routine to accommodate your changing body, you can stay active and healthy throughout your pregnancy. Remember to prioritize safety, listen to your body, and make adjustments as needed to ensure a positive and enjoyable experience.

Exercise and Pregnancy Trimester

As your body changes with each passing trimester, it's essential to adapt your workout routines accordingly. Each trimester brings unique physical and hormonal changes that can affect your exercise capacity and comfort levels. This section provides trimester-specific exercise guidelines to help you stay active and healthy throughout your pregnancy.

First Trimester (Weeks 1-12):

During the first trimester, your body undergoes significant changes as it adapts to pregnancy. Morning sickness, fatigue, and hormonal fluctuations are common during this period. While it may be challenging to stay active, gentle exercises can help alleviate some of these symptoms and set the foundation for a healthy pregnancy.

1. Listen to Your Body: Fatigue and nausea may affect your ability to exercise. Listen to your body and take it easy if you're not feeling well. Gentle activities like walking, stretching, and prenatal yoga can be beneficial.

2. Focus on Low-Impact Activities: Engage in low-impact exercises such as walking, swimming, and stationary cycling. These activities are gentle on your joints and can help improve energy levels without putting excessive strain on your body.

3. Avoid High-Risk Activities: Avoid activities that carry a risk of falling or abdominal trauma, such as skiing, horseback riding, and contact sports. These activities can pose a serious risk to both you and your baby.

4. Stay Hydrated and Nourished: Drink plenty of water before, during, and after exercise to stay hydrated. Eat small, frequent meals to maintain energy levels and reduce nausea.

Second Trimester (Weeks 13-26):

The second trimester is often considered the "golden period" of pregnancy, as many women experience a reduction in morning sickness and an increase in energy levels. This is an excellent time to engage in regular physical activity and strengthen your body for the months ahead.

1. Maintain a Regular Exercise Routine: With increased energy levels, you can maintain a regular exercise routine. Aim for at least 30 minutes of moderate-intensity exercise most days of the week.

2. Focus on Strengthening Exercises: Incorporate strength training exercises to build muscle and improve overall fitness. Focus on exercises that strengthen the core, back, and pelvic floor muscles. Use light weights or resistance bands for added resistance.

3. Modify Exercises for Comfort: As your belly grows, certain exercises may become uncomfortable. Modify exercises to accommodate your changing body. For example, switch from traditional abdominal exercises to side-lying or seated exercises that target the core.

4. Stay Cool and Hydrated: Exercise in a cool environment and wear loose, breathable clothing to prevent overheating. Continue to stay hydrated by drinking plenty of water.

Third Trimester (Weeks 27-40):

In the third trimester, your body is preparing for labor and delivery. Physical changes such as increased weight, swelling, and fatigue can make exercise more challenging. However, staying active can help manage these discomforts and prepare your body for childbirth.

1. Engage in Gentle Activities: Focus on gentle activities like walking, swimming, and prenatal yoga. These exercises can help alleviate back pain, reduce swelling, and improve circulation.

2. Practice Pelvic Floor Exercises: Continue to perform pelvic floor exercises (Kegels) to strengthen the muscles needed for labor and delivery. Strong pelvic floor muscles can also aid in postpartum recovery.

3. Avoid High-Impact and High-Risk Activities: Avoid high-impact activities and exercises that require lying flat on your back, as this can compress the vena cava and reduce blood flow to your baby. Opt for seated or side-lying exercises instead.

4. Listen to Your Body: Pay close attention to your body's signals and adjust your exercise routine as needed. If you experience any pain, dizziness, or shortness of breath, stop exercising and consult your healthcare provider.

By following these trimester-specific exercise guidelines, you can stay active and healthy throughout your pregnancy. Remember to prioritize safety, listen to your body, and make adjustments as needed to ensure a positive and enjoyable experience.

Getting Started and Staying Motivated

Beginning an exercise regime may seem daunting, especially when grappling with nausea, heartburn, or fatigue common in pregnancy. However, with the right approach and mindset, you can overcome these barriers and establish a consistent and enjoyable exercise routine. This section provides practical advice on getting started, setting realistic goals, and staying motivated throughout your pregnancy.

Finding Prenatal Exercise Classes or Online Resources:

1. Local Prenatal Classes: Many communities offer prenatal exercise classes such as prenatal yoga, Pilates, and water aerobics. These classes are specifically designed for pregnant women and provide a safe and supportive environment. Check with local gyms, community centers, and hospitals for available classes.

2. Online Resources: If you prefer exercising at home, numerous online resources offer prenatal workout videos and programs. Websites, apps, and streaming services provide a wide range of options, from yoga and Pilates to strength training and cardio workouts. Look for certified prenatal instructors to ensure the exercises are safe and appropriate for pregnancy.

Setting Realistic Goals and Creating a Workout Schedule:

1. Start Slow and Build Gradually: If you were not active before pregnancy, start with short, low-intensity workouts and gradually increase the duration and intensity as your fitness improves. Aim for at least 30 minutes of moderate-intensity exercise most days of the week.
2. Set Specific, Achievable Goal: Set specific and achievable goals to keep yourself motivated. For example, aim to complete a certain number of workouts per week or gradually increase the duration of your walks. Celebrate your progress and achievements, no matter how small.
3. Create a Flexible Workout Schedule: Create a workout schedule that fits your lifestyle and energy levels. Be flexible and adjust your schedule as needed, considering your physical and emotional state. Consistency is key, but it's also important to listen to your body and rest when necessary.

Tips for Staying Motivated and Overcoming Barriers to Exercise:

1. Find a Workout Buddy: Exercising with a friend or partner can make workouts more enjoyable and hold you accountable. Consider joining a prenatal exercise class or forming a walking group with other pregnant women.
2. Make Exercise Enjoyable: Choose activities that you enjoy and look forward to. Whether it's dancing, swimming, or taking a scenic walk, finding joy in your workouts will help you stay committed.
3. Track Your Progress: Keep a workout journal or use a fitness app to track your progress. Seeing your achievements can boost motivation and help you stay on track with your fitness goals.
4. Stay Positive and Patient: Understand that pregnancy comes with its own set of challenges, and it's okay to have days when you don't feel like exercising. Stay positive and patient with yourself, and focus on the long-term benefits of staying active.
5. Incorporate Exercise into Daily Routine: Find ways to incorporate physical activity into your daily routine. Take the stairs instead of the elevator, park farther away from your destination, or take short breaks to stretch and move around.
6. Seek Support and Encouragement: Share your fitness goals with your partner, friends, and family. Their support and encouragement can make a significant difference in staying motivated and committed to your exercise routine.

By finding the right resources, setting realistic goals, and staying motivated, you can establish a consistent and enjoyable exercise routine that benefits both you and your baby. Remember, the journey towards a healthy and active pregnancy is unique for every woman. Embrace the process, listen to your body, and celebrate your progress along the way.

In this chapter, we explored the importance of staying active and healthy during pregnancy, providing practical tips, safety guidelines, and motivational advice to help you maintain an active lifestyle.

Key Takeaways:

- ❖ Active and Healthy Physical Activity: We discussed the myriad benefits of exercise during pregnancy, including improved mood and energy levels, better sleep, reduced pregnancy discomforts, and preparation for labor and delivery. Safety guidelines and precautions were emphasized to ensure the well-being of both mother and baby.

- ❖ Special Considerations: Modifying Your Routine: Adjusting exercise intensity and frequency, avoiding high-impact activities and contact sports, and incorporating pelvic floor exercises and stretching were highlighted as essential strategies for maintaining a safe and effective exercise routine.

- ❖ Exercise and Pregnancy Trimester: Trimester-specific exercise guidelines were provided, helping you adapt your workout routines to the unique changes and challenges of each stage of pregnancy. By following these guidelines, you can stay active and comfortable throughout your pregnancy journey.

- ❖ Getting Started and Staying Motivated: Practical advice on finding prenatal exercise classes or online resources, setting realistic goals, creating a workout schedule, and staying motivated was shared to help you overcome barriers and establish a consistent exercise routine.

As you continue your pregnancy journey, remember to listen to your body, stay hydrated, and seek support from healthcare professionals for personalized guidance. Every step you take towards staying active and healthy contributes to the well-being of both you and your baby.

Chapter 7:

Managing Discomforts

Pregnancy is a transformative journey, filled with a mix of emotions ranging from joy and excitement to anxiety and uncertainty. As your body nurtures new life, it undergoes a multitude of changes that can sometimes lead to discomfort. Understanding and managing these discomforts is crucial for maintaining both your physical and mental well-being. In this chapter, we'll delve into the most common pregnancy-related discomforts and provide you with practical strategies to alleviate them, ensuring you can enjoy this special time to the fullest.

Pregnancy discomforts vary widely from one woman to another. Some may experience mild inconveniences, while others might face more severe challenges. Regardless of the intensity, acknowledging these discomforts and knowing how to manage them effectively can make a significant difference in your overall pregnancy experience. From the queasiness of morning sickness to the aches of back pain and the restlessness of insomnia, we'll cover a broad spectrum of issues that many pregnant women encounter.

We'll explore natural remedies like herbal teas and essential oils, discuss lifestyle changes including posture correction and stress management, and provide guidelines on when to seek medical attention for severe discomforts. Additionally, we'll highlight self-care practices that promote emotional well-being, as maintaining a positive mindset is just as important as physical comfort during pregnancy.

By the end of this chapter, you'll be equipped with a comprehensive understanding of various pregnancy discomforts and a toolkit of strategies to manage them. Our goal is to support you in navigating these challenges with confidence and ease, helping you to embrace this beautiful journey with a sense of empowerment and serenity. So, let's embark on this path together, ensuring your pregnancy is as comfortable and nourished as possible.

Morning Sickness

Morning sickness, characterized by nausea and vomiting, affects up to 80% of pregnant women, especially during the first trimester. Despite its name, morning sickness can occur at any time of the day or night. The exact cause is not fully understood, but it is believed to be related to the rapid increase in hormones, such as human chorionic gonadotropin (hCG) and estrogen, during early pregnancy.

Causes:
- Hormonal changes: Elevated levels of hCG and estrogen.
- Increased sensitivity to odors.
- Low blood sugar levels.

Genetic factors: A family history of morning sickness.

Relief Measures and Management Strategies:

Dietary Adjustments:
Eat small, frequent meals throughout the day to keep your blood sugar levels stable.
Avoid foods and smells that trigger nausea. Opt for bland, easy-to-digest foods like crackers, toast, and bananas.
Keep a snack, such as crackers, by your bedside to eat before getting out of bed in the morning.
Stay hydrated by sipping water, ginger ale, or herbal teas throughout the day. Avoid drinking large amounts at once.
Ginger:
Ginger has natural anti-nausea properties. Try ginger tea, ginger ale, or ginger candies to help soothe your stomach.
Incorporate fresh ginger into your meals or consume ginger supplements after consulting your healthcare provider.
Vitamin B6:
Vitamin B6 supplements have been shown to reduce nausea in some pregnant women. Discuss with your healthcare provider the appropriate dosage for you.
Acupressure:
Wristbands that apply pressure to the P6 acupressure point on your inner wrist can help alleviate nausea. These are often used for motion sickness and can be effective for morning sickness as well.
Rest and Relaxation:
Fatigue can exacerbate nausea, so ensure you get plenty of rest.
Practice relaxation techniques such as deep breathing, meditation, or prenatal yoga to reduce stress and promote overall well-being.
Medical Intervention:

In severe cases, where vomiting is frequent and intense, leading to dehydration and weight loss, medical intervention may be necessary. Prescription medications such as antihistamines, antiemetic, or antacids may be recommended by your healthcare provider.

Lifestyle Tips:

Keep your living space well-ventilated to avoid strong odors.

Wear comfortable, loose-fitting clothes to prevent any pressure on your stomach.

Avoid lying down immediately after eating to prevent acid reflux and further nausea.

Morning sickness can be challenging, but it usually subsides by the second trimester. By implementing these strategies and seeking support when needed, you can manage this discomfort effectively and focus on the joy and excitement of your pregnancy journey.

Heartburn

Heartburn is a common discomfort during pregnancy, affecting many expectant mothers, especially in the later stages. It is characterized by a burning sensation in the chest or throat, often accompanied by a sour or bitter taste in the mouth. This discomfort is caused by stomach acid flowing back into the esophagus, which can be exacerbated by the physical and hormonal changes occurring during pregnancy.

Causes:

- Hormonal changes: Increased levels of progesterone relax the valve between the stomach and esophagus, allowing stomach acid to escape.
- Physical pressure: As the uterus expands, it pushes the stomach upward, increasing the likelihood of acid reflux.
- Slow digestion: Pregnancy hormones can slow down the digestive process, causing food to remain in the stomach longer and increasing the risk of heartburn.

Relief Measures and Management Strategies:

Dietary Adjustments:

Eat smaller, more frequent meals rather than three large meals a day to prevent the stomach from becoming too full.

Avoid trigger foods such as spicy, fatty, or acidic foods, which can exacerbate heartburn. Common culprits include chocolate, caffeine, citrus fruits, tomatoes, and fried foods.

Stay upright after eating. Wait at least one hour before lying down to allow time for digestion.

Chew gum after meals to increase saliva production, which can help neutralize stomach acid.

Hydration:

Drink plenty of water throughout the day, but avoid drinking large amounts during meals to prevent overfilling the stomach.

Sipping on herbal teas, such as ginger or chamomile, can help soothe the digestive tract.

Clothing:

Wear loose-fitting clothes to avoid putting additional pressure on your stomach and lower esophagus.

Sleeping Position:

Elevate the head of your bed by placing blocks under the legs or using a wedge pillow. This helps keep stomach acid down during the night.

Sleep on your left side to reduce the likelihood of acid reflux, as this position helps keep the stomach below the esophagus.

Over-the-Counter Remedies:

Antacids can provide quick relief by neutralizing stomach acid. However, consult your healthcare provider before taking any medication to ensure it is safe for use during pregnancy.

H2 blockers or proton pump inhibitors may be recommended for more severe cases, but these should only be used under medical supervision.

Lifestyle Tips:

Avoid eating close to bedtime to reduce the risk of nighttime heartburn.

Practice stress-reducing activities such as prenatal yoga, meditation, or gentle exercise, as stress can worsen heartburn.

Keep a food diary to identify and avoid specific foods that trigger your heartburn.

By making these adjustments and being mindful of your habits, you can effectively manage heartburn during pregnancy and minimize discomfort. If heartburn persists or becomes severe, consult your healthcare provider for further guidance and treatment options.

Fatigue

Fatigue is a common and often overwhelming experience during pregnancy. As your body works tirelessly to support the growing life within you, it's natural to feel more tired than usual. Fatigue can occur at any stage of pregnancy but is especially prevalent during the first and third trimesters.

Causes:

- Hormonal changes: Increased levels of progesterone can make you feel sleepy and sluggish.

- Increased blood volume: Your body is producing more blood to support your baby, which requires extra energy.
- Emotional stress: Anxiety and stress about the pregnancy and impending parenthood can contribute to fatigue.
- Physical demands: As your baby grows, your body works harder to support the added weight, which can lead to exhaustion.
- Sleep disturbances: Discomfort, frequent trips to the bathroom, and vivid dreams can disrupt sleep patterns.

Relief Measures and Management Strategies:

Rest and Sleep:
Prioritize sleep and aim for 7-9 hours per night. Take short naps during the day if needed, but try to keep them under 30 minutes to avoid interfering with nighttime sleep.
Create a relaxing bedtime routine to signal your body that it's time to wind down. This might include reading a book, taking a warm bath, or practicing gentle stretching.
Ensure your sleeping environment is comfortable. Use pillows to support your body and invest in a good mattress if necessary.
Nutrition:
Eat a balanced diet rich in iron, protein, and complex carbohydrates to maintain energy levels. Include foods like lean meats, leafy greens, whole grains, and legumes.
Stay hydrated by drinking plenty of water throughout the day. Dehydration can exacerbate feelings of fatigue.
Avoid excessive caffeine and sugar, which can cause energy spikes and crashes.
Physical Activity:
Engage in regular, moderate exercise such as walking, swimming, or prenatal yoga. Exercise can boost energy levels, improve mood, and promote better sleep.
Listen to your body and avoid overexertion. It's important to find a balance between staying active and getting enough rest.
Stress Management:
Practice relaxation techniques such as deep breathing, meditation, or mindfulness to reduce stress and promote a sense of calm.
Consider joining a prenatal yoga or meditation class to learn techniques specifically tailored for pregnant women.
Support System:
Seek support from your partner, family, and friends. Don't hesitate to ask for help with daily tasks to conserve your energy.

Consider joining a pregnancy support group to connect with other expectant mothers who can share their experiences and provide encouragement.

Medical Advice:

If fatigue is severe or persistent, consult your healthcare provider. They can check for underlying conditions such as anemia or thyroid issues that might be contributing to your exhaustion.

By prioritizing rest, maintaining a balanced diet, staying active, and managing stress, you can effectively combat pregnancy-related fatigue. Remember to listen to your body and give yourself permission to rest when needed. Taking care of yourself is essential for both your well-being and the healthy development of your baby.

Back Pain

Back pain is a common complaint during pregnancy, affecting many women as their bodies adjust to the growing baby. The pain can range from a dull ache to sharp discomfort and is typically experienced in the lower back. This discomfort is often due to a combination of hormonal changes, weight gain, and postural adjustments.

Causes:

- Hormonal changes: The hormone relaxin, which helps prepare your body for childbirth, loosens ligaments and joints, making your back more prone to pain.
- Weight gain: As your baby grows, the added weight increases the stress on your back muscles and spine.
- Posture changes: The expanding belly shifts your center of gravity, leading to changes in posture and increased strain on your back.
- Muscle separation: The growing uterus can cause the rectus abdominis muscles to separate, weakening the core and placing more pressure on the back

Relief Measures and Management Strategies:

Exercise:

Engage in regular, low-impact exercise to strengthen your back and abdominal muscles. Activities like walking, swimming, and prenatal yoga can be particularly beneficial.

Perform specific exercises designed to strengthen the core and improve posture, such as pelvic tilts and cat-cow stretches.

Posture:

Be mindful of your posture when standing, sitting, and walking. Keep your shoulders back and avoid slouching.

Use a chair with good lumbar support, or place a small pillow behind your lower back when sitting.

Lifting Techniques:

Avoid heavy lifting whenever possible. If you must lift something, bend at your knees and keep your back straight to minimize strain.

Supportive Gear:

Wear comfortable, supportive shoes with low heels and good arch support to reduce strain on your back.

Consider using a maternity support belt to help distribute the weight of your growing belly and provide extra support for your back.

Sleep Position:

Sleep on your side with a pillow between your knees to support proper spinal alignment. This can help relieve pressure on your back.

Use additional pillows to support your belly and back, ensuring a comfortable sleeping position.

Heat and Cold Therapy:

Apply a warm compress or heating pad to your lower back to soothe sore muscles. Be cautious with heat application to avoid overheating.

Use a cold pack or ice wrapped in a towel to reduce inflammation and numb the area if the pain is acute.

Massage and Chiropractic Care:

Prenatal massages can help relax tight muscles and alleviate back pain. Seek a certified prenatal massage therapist for safe and effective treatment.

Consult with a chiropractor who specializes in prenatal care for adjustments that can help relieve back pain and improve alignment.

By incorporating these strategies into your daily routine, you can manage and alleviate back pain during pregnancy. Remember to listen to your body and take breaks when needed. If back pain persists or becomes severe, consult your healthcare provider for further evaluation and treatment options.

Sciatica

Sciatica is a condition characterized by pain radiating along the sciatic nerve, which runs from the lower back through the hips and down each leg. During pregnancy, the expanding uterus and the added weight can put pressure on this nerve, leading to discomfort and pain.

Causes:

- Uterine pressure: As the uterus grows, it can press on the sciatic nerve, causing pain.
- Postural changes: The shift in your center of gravity and changes in posture can contribute to sciatic nerve compression.
- Muscle tension: Tight muscles in the buttocks and lower back can irritate the sciatic nerve.

Relief Measures and Management Strategies:

Stretching Exercises:
Gentle stretching exercises can help relieve tension and pressure on the sciatic nerve. Focus on stretches that target the lower back, hips, and legs.
Examples include the piriformis stretch, seated forward bend, and cat-cow stretch.
Prenatal Yoga:
Prenatal yoga can improve flexibility, strengthen muscles, and promote better posture. Many yoga poses specifically target areas that can help alleviate sciatic pain.
Poses such as the child's pose, pigeon pose, and the bridge pose can be particularly beneficial.
Heat and Cold Therapy:
Apply a warm compress or heating pad to the lower back and buttocks to relax muscles and reduce pain.
Use an ice pack on the affected area to reduce inflammation and numb the pain.
Massage Therapy:
Prenatal massages can help relax tight muscles and reduce sciatic pain. Seek a certified prenatal massage therapist for safe and effective treatment.
Focus on the lower back, hips, and legs during the massage.
Physical Activity:
Engage in regular, low-impact exercises such as walking, swimming, and water aerobics. These activities can help strengthen muscles and reduce pressure on the sciatic nerve.
Avoid activities that involve heavy lifting or high impact, as they can exacerbate sciatic pain.
Posture and Body Mechanics:
Maintain good posture while sitting, standing, and walking to reduce pressure on the sciatic nerve.
Use a chair with proper lumbar support and avoid sitting for extended periods. If you must sit for long periods, take regular breaks to stand and stretch.
Sleep Position:

Sleep on your side with a pillow between your knees to keep your spine aligned and reduce pressure on the sciatic nerve.

Use additional pillows to support your belly and back for a more comfortable sleeping position.

Medical Consultation:

If sciatic pain is severe or persistent, consult your healthcare provider. They may recommend physical therapy or other treatments to help manage the pain.

By incorporating these strategies into your routine, you can alleviate sciatic pain and improve your overall comfort during pregnancy. Remember to listen to your body and take breaks when needed. If sciatic pain persists or worsens, seek medical advice for further evaluation and treatment options.

Braxton Hicks Contractions

Braxton Hicks contractions, often referred to as "false labor," are irregular and usually painless contractions that can occur throughout pregnancy, particularly in the third trimester. These contractions are the body's way of preparing for actual labor, but they do not indicate that labor is imminent.

Causes:

- Uterine muscle practice: The uterus contracts intermittently to prepare for the intense contractions of labor.
- Dehydration: Lack of adequate hydration can trigger Braxton Hicks contractions.
- Physical activity: Vigorous exercise or physical exertion can cause these contractions.
- Full bladder: A full bladder can sometimes lead to Braxton Hicks contractions.
- Sexual activity: Orgasm can trigger uterine contractions, which are typically Braxton Hicks.

Relief Measures and Management Strategies:

Hydration:

Drink plenty of water throughout the day to stay hydrated. Dehydration can trigger or worsen Braxton Hicks contractions.

Keep a water bottle with you to ensure you're sipping water regularly.

Rest and Relaxation:

If you experience Braxton Hicks contractions after physical activity, rest for a while. Sit down, put your feet up, and relax until the contractions subside.

Practice relaxation techniques such as deep breathing, meditation, or prenatal yoga to help your body and mind relax.

Change Positions:

Sometimes changing your position can help relieve Braxton Hicks contractions. If you've been sitting for a while, stand up and walk around. If you've been active, try lying down on your side.

Warm Bath:

Taking a warm bath can help relax your muscles and reduce the frequency and intensity of Braxton Hicks contractions.

Ensure the water is warm, not hot, to avoid overheating

Empty your Bladder:

A full bladder can sometimes trigger Braxton Hicks contractions. Make sure to empty your bladder regularly.

Avoid Overexertion:

While staying active is important, avoid overexerting yourself. Listen to your body and take breaks as needed.

Engage in moderate, low-impact exercises such as walking or prenatal yoga rather than high-intensity workouts.

Medical Advice:

If you're unsure whether the contractions you're experiencing are Braxton Hicks or actual labor contractions, contact your healthcare provider for guidance.

If the contractions become regular, increase in intensity, or are accompanied by other signs of labor such as back pain, pressure, or fluid leakage, seek medical attention immediately.

Understanding Braxton Hicks contractions and learning to differentiate them from actual labor contractions can help ease anxiety and ensure you're prepared for when true labor begins. By staying hydrated, resting when needed, and practicing relaxation techniques, you can manage these contractions and remain comfortable throughout your pregnancy.

Varicose Veins

Varicose veins are swollen, twisted veins that often appear on the legs during pregnancy. They occur due to the increased blood volume and the pressure of the growing uterus on the veins in the lower body. While generally harmless, varicose veins can be uncomfortable and sometimes painful.

Causes:

- Increased blood volume: During pregnancy, blood volume increases to support the growing baby, which can cause veins to enlarge.
- Hormonal changes: Pregnancy hormones, particularly progesterone, relax the walls of blood vessels, making them more prone to swelling.
- Pressure from the uterus: As the uterus expands, it puts pressure on the inferior vena cava (the large vein that carries blood from the lower body to the heart) and pelvic veins, slowing blood flow from the legs.
- Family history: A genetic predisposition to varicose veins can increase your likelihood of developing them during pregnancy.

Relief Measures and Management Strategies:

Exercise:

Regular, moderate exercise such as walking, swimming, or prenatal yoga can improve circulation and reduce the risk of varicose veins.

Avoid standing or sitting for long periods. Take breaks to move around and stretch your legs.

Elevate Your Legs:

Elevate your legs whenever possible to improve blood flow back to the heart. Prop your legs up on a pillow or use a footstool when sitting.

Lie down with your legs elevated above heart level for short periods throughout the day to reduce swelling.

Compression Stockings:

Wear compression stockings to support your veins and improve circulation. These stockings apply gentle pressure to your legs, helping blood flow back to your heart.

Put on compression stockings in the morning before you get out of bed, when your veins are less swollen.

Avoid Crossing Your Legs:

Avoid sitting with your legs crossed, as this can restrict blood flow and increase pressure on your veins.

Sleep Position:

Sleep on your left side to reduce pressure on the inferior vena cava and improve blood flow from the lower body.

Use a pregnancy pillow to support your body and maintain a comfortable sleeping position.

Weight Management:

Maintain a healthy weight to reduce pressure on your veins. Follow a balanced diet and stay active to manage weight gain during pregnancy.

Clothing:

Wear loose-fitting clothes that do not restrict circulation, especially around your waist, legs, and groin.

Hydration and Diet:

Drink plenty of water to stay hydrated and support healthy blood flow.

Eat a diet rich in fiber to prevent constipation, which can exacerbate varicose veins. Include fruits, vegetables, whole grains, and legumes in your meals.

Medical Consultation:

If varicose veins become painful, swollen, or inflamed, consult your healthcare provider. They may recommend additional treatments or refer you to a specialist.

Post-pregnancy, if varicose veins persist or cause significant discomfort, there are medical procedures available to treat them.

By incorporating these strategies into your daily routine, you can manage and alleviate the discomfort associated with varicose veins during pregnancy. Remember to stay active, elevate your legs, and use compression stockings to support your veins and improve circulation. If symptoms persist or worsen, seek medical advice for further evaluation and treatment options.

Hemorrhoids

Hemorrhoids are swollen veins in the rectal area that can cause discomfort, itching, and bleeding. They are common during pregnancy due to increased pressure on the veins in the pelvis and rectum, as well as hormonal changes that can cause veins to swell.

Causes:

- Increased blood volume: The increased blood volume during pregnancy can cause veins to enlarge, including those in the rectal area.
- Pressure from the uterus: The growing uterus puts pressure on the veins in the pelvis and lower rectum, contributing to the development of hemorrhoids.
- Constipation: Pregnancy hormones can slow down the digestive system, leading to constipation and straining during bowel movements, which can cause hemorrhoids.
- Hormonal changes: Hormones such as progesterone relax the walls of blood vessels, making them more prone to swelling.

Relief Measures and Management Strategies:

Hydration and Diet:

Drink plenty of water throughout the day to stay hydrated and prevent constipation.

Eat a high-fiber diet, including fruits, vegetables, whole grains, and legumes, to promote regular bowel movements and reduce straining.

Avoid Straining:

Avoid straining during bowel movements, as this can exacerbate hemorrhoids. If you experience constipation, use stool softeners or fiber supplements as recommended by your healthcare provider.

Bathroom Habits:

Go to the bathroom as soon as you feel the urge to have a bowel movement. Delaying can lead to harder stools and increased straining.

Use unscented, gentle wipes instead of toilet paper to clean the rectal area after bowel movements to reduce irritation.

Warm Baths:

Take warm baths or sitz baths (sitting in a shallow bath of warm water) to soothe and reduce the swelling of hemorrhoids. Do this for 15-20 minutes several times a day.

Cold Compresses:

Apply cold compresses or ice packs to the affected area to reduce swelling and provide relief from pain and itching. Use a clean cloth to wrap the ice pack and apply it for 10-15 minutes.

Topical Treatments:

Use over-the-counter hemorrhoid creams or ointments to relieve pain, itching, and swelling. Consult your healthcare provider before using any medication during pregnancy.

Witch hazel pads can also provide soothing relief from hemorrhoid symptoms.

Avoid Prolonged Sitting:

Avoid sitting for long periods, as this can increase pressure on the rectal veins. Take breaks to stand up and move around regularly.

Sleep Position:

Sleep on your side to reduce pressure on the rectal veins and improve blood flow.

Medical Consultation:

If hemorrhoids become very painful, bleed excessively, or do not improve with home treatments, consult your healthcare provider. They may recommend additional treatments or refer you to a specialist.

By following these strategies, you can manage and alleviate the discomfort associated with hemorrhoids during pregnancy. Focus on hydration, a high-fiber diet, gentle bathroom habits, and soothing treatments to find relief. If symptoms persist or worsen, seek medical advice for further evaluation and treatment options.

Restless leg syndrome (RLS) is a condition characterized by an uncontrollable urge to move the legs, often accompanied by uncomfortable sensations such as tingling, itching, or aching. RLS can be particularly bothersome during pregnancy, especially in the third trimester, and can interfere with sleep.

Causes:

- Hormonal changes: Pregnancy-related hormonal fluctuations, particularly increased levels of estrogen, can contribute to RLS.
- Iron deficiency: Low levels of iron in the blood, common during pregnancy, can exacerbate RLS symptoms.
- Circulation changes: The increased blood volume and changes in circulation during pregnancy can affect nerve function and contribute to RLS.
- Genetics: A family history of RLS can increase the likelihood of experiencing the condition during pregnancy.

Relief Measures and Management Strategies:

Iron and Nutrient Intake:
Ensure adequate intake of iron-rich foods, such as lean meats, leafy greens, legumes, and fortified cereals. Iron supplements may also be recommended by your healthcare provider if necessary.
Include foods rich in folate, magnesium, and vitamin B12 in your diet, as deficiencies in these nutrients can also contribute to RLS.
Regular Exercise:
Engage in regular, moderate exercise such as walking, swimming, or prenatal yoga to improve circulation and reduce RLS symptoms.
Avoid vigorous exercise close to bedtime, as it can sometimes exacerbate symptoms.
Sleep Hygiene:
Establish a consistent sleep routine by going to bed and waking up at the same time each day.
Create a relaxing bedtime routine that includes activities such as reading, taking a warm bath, or practicing gentle stretches.
Leg Massages and Stretches:
Massage your legs before bed to relax muscles and reduce RLS symptoms. Use gentle, circular motions and consider using a soothing lotion or oil.

Perform leg stretches before bed to alleviate tension and discomfort. Focus on stretches that target the calves, hamstrings, and feet.

Warm and Cold Therapy:

Alternate between warm and cold compresses on your legs to soothe muscles and improve circulation.

Take a warm bath before bed to relax your muscles and prepare your body for sleep.

Avoid Triggers:

Limit caffeine intake, as it can exacerbate RLS symptoms. Avoid coffee, tea, chocolate, and certain sodas, especially in the afternoon and evening.

Reduce stress and anxiety through relaxation techniques such as deep breathing, meditation, or prenatal yoga.

Comfortable Sleeping Environment:

Ensure your sleeping environment is comfortable and conducive to sleep. Use supportive pillows, maintain a cool room temperature, and reduce noise and light disturbances.

Medical Consultation:

If RLS symptoms are severe or persistent, consult your healthcare provider. They can assess your nutrient levels and recommend appropriate supplements or treatments.

In some cases, medication may be prescribed to manage RLS symptoms. Always follow your healthcare provider's guidance and recommendations.

By incorporating these strategies into your daily routine, you can manage and alleviate the discomfort associated with restless leg syndrome during pregnancy. Focus on maintaining a balanced diet, regular exercise, and good sleep hygiene to find relief. If symptoms persist or worsen, seek medical advice for further evaluation and treatment options.

Insomnia

Insomnia, or difficulty falling and staying asleep, is a common issue during pregnancy. Hormonal changes, physical discomfort, and anxiety can all contribute to disrupted sleep. Managing insomnia is crucial for maintaining overall health and well-being during pregnancy.

Causes:

- Hormonal changes: Pregnancy hormones, particularly progesterone, can affect sleep patterns and lead to insomnia.
- Physical discomfort: As the pregnancy progresses, physical discomforts such as back pain, frequent urination, and restless leg syndrome can disrupt sleep.
- Anxiety and stress: Worries about pregnancy, childbirth, and parenting can contribute to insomnia.

- Frequent urination: The growing uterus puts pressure on the bladder, leading to increased nighttime trips to the bathroom.

Relief Measures and Management Strategies:
Establish a Bedtime Routine:
Create a consistent bedtime routine to signal your body that it's time to wind down. This can include activities such as reading, taking a warm bath, or practicing relaxation exercises.
Go to bed and wake up at the same time every day to regulate your sleep-wake cycle.
Create a Comfortable Sleep Environment:
Ensure your bedroom is cool, dark, and quiet. Use blackout curtains, earplugs, or a white noise machine if necessary.
Invest in a comfortable mattress and supportive pillows. Consider using a pregnancy pillow to support your body and reduce discomfort.
Limit Screen Time:
Avoid screens (phones, tablets, computers, and TVs) at least an hour before bed, as the blue light emitted can interfere with your body's production of melatonin, a hormone that regulates sleep.
Practice Relaxation Techniques:
Engage in relaxation techniques such as deep breathing, meditation, or prenatal yoga to reduce stress and prepare your body for sleep.
Progressive muscle relaxation, where you tense and then release each muscle group in your body, can also help promote relaxation.
Monitor Your Diet:
Avoid caffeine and large meals close to bedtime, as they can interfere with sleep. Opt for a light snack if you're hungry before bed.
Drink plenty of water throughout the day, but reduce fluid intake in the evening to minimize nighttime bathroom trips.
Stay Active:
Regular, moderate exercise such as walking, swimming, or prenatal yoga can improve sleep quality. Aim for at least 30 minutes of activity most days of the week.
Avoid vigorous exercise close to bedtime, as it can sometimes have a stimulating effect.
Manage Stress and Anxiety:
Address any worries or anxieties by talking to a supportive friend, partner, or counselor. Writing down your thoughts in a journal can also help clear your mind before bed.
Consider attending prenatal classes to prepare for childbirth and parenting, which can alleviate some of your concerns.
Limit Naps:

While napping can be beneficial, avoid long or late-afternoon naps that can interfere with nighttime sleep.

Medical Consultation:

If insomnia persists or significantly impacts your daily life, consult your healthcare provider. They can help identify any underlying issues and recommend appropriate treatments or therapies.

In some cases, medication or supplements may be prescribed to improve sleep. Always follow your healthcare provider's guidance and recommendations.

By incorporating these strategies into your routine, you can manage and alleviate the discomfort associated with insomnia during pregnancy. Focus on establishing a consistent bedtime routine, creating a comfortable sleep environment, and practicing relaxation techniques to improve your sleep quality. If symptoms persist or worsen, seek medical advice for further evaluation and treatment options.

Natural Remedies for Common Discomforts

Pregnancy discomforts can often be managed with natural remedies that provide relief without the use of medications. Herbal teas and essential oils are popular choices among expectant mothers seeking natural alternatives. These remedies can help alleviate a variety of symptoms and promote overall well-being.

Herbal Teas:

Ginger Tea:

Ginger tea is renowned for its ability to combat nausea and vomiting, making it a popular choice for morning sickness relief. It can also aid digestion and reduce inflammation.

To prepare, steep a few slices of fresh ginger in hot water for 10-15 minutes. Add honey and lemon for extra flavor and benefits.

Peppermint Tea:

Peppermint tea can soothe an upset stomach and alleviate bloating and gas. It also has a calming effect, which can help reduce stress and anxiety.

Steep peppermint leaves in hot water for 5-10 minutes. Drink it warm or cool, depending on your preference.

Chamomile Tea:
Chamomile tea is known for its calming properties and can help promote better sleep. It can also relieve mild digestive issues and reduce inflammation.
Steep chamomile flowers in hot water for 5-10 minutes. Drink it before bed to help with insomnia.
Raspberry Leaf Tea:
Raspberry leaf tea is often used in the third trimester to tone the uterus and prepare for labor. It can also help with nausea and improve digestion.
Steep raspberry leaves in hot water for 10-15 minutes. Consult your healthcare provider before using raspberry leaf tea, especially in early pregnancy.

Essential Oils:

Lavender Oil:
Lavender oil is known for its relaxing and calming properties. It can help with anxiety, stress, and insomnia.
Add a few drops of lavender oil to a diffuser or a warm bath. You can also mix it with a carrier oil (such as coconut or almond oil) and use it for a gentle massage.
Peppermint Oil:
Peppermint oil can alleviate headaches, reduce nausea, and improve energy levels.
Inhale the scent directly from the bottle or use a diffuser. For headaches, dilute with a carrier oil and apply to the temples and neck.
Eucalyptus Oil:
Eucalyptus oil can help with respiratory issues, such as congestion and colds. It also has anti-inflammatory properties.
Add a few drops to a diffuser or a bowl of hot water and inhale the steam. You can also mix it with a carrier oil and apply it to the chest.
Ginger Oil:
Ginger oil is effective in reducing nausea and improving digestion.
Use a diffuser to inhale the scent or mix with a carrier oil and massage onto the stomach.
Safety Considerations:
Always dilute essential oils with a carrier oil before applying them to the skin to avoid irritation.
Consult with your healthcare provider before using any herbal teas or essential oils, especially if you have any pre-existing conditions or are taking other medications.
Avoid certain essential oils that are not safe for use during pregnancy, such as clary sage, rosemary, and cinnamon.

Use herbal teas and essential oils in moderation. While they are natural, excessive use can still cause adverse effects.
Lifestyle Changes:

Hydration:
Drink plenty of water throughout the day to stay hydrated and support overall health. Proper hydration can help with a variety of pregnancy-related discomforts, such as constipation and swelling.
Balanced Diet:
Maintain a balanced diet rich in fruits, vegetables, whole grains, and lean proteins. Proper nutrition supports overall health and can help prevent or alleviate many common pregnancy discomforts.
Regular Exercise:
Engage in regular, moderate exercise such as walking, swimming, or prenatal yoga. Exercise can improve circulation, reduce stress, and alleviate symptoms like back pain and constipation.
Rest and Relaxation:

Prioritize rest and relaxation to manage stress and promote overall well-being. Practice relaxation techniques such as deep breathing, meditation, or prenatal yoga.
Incorporating natural remedies and lifestyle changes into your daily routine can help manage and alleviate common pregnancy discomforts. By using herbal teas and essential oils safely and maintaining a healthy lifestyle, you can enhance your overall well-being during pregnancy. Always consult with your healthcare provider before starting any new remedies or making significant lifestyle changes.

Lifestyle Changes for Managing Pregnancy Discomforts

During pregnancy, adopting certain lifestyle changes can significantly reduce discomforts and enhance overall well-being. By making simple adjustments to daily habits, expectant mothers can manage common pregnancy-related issues effectively.

   1. **Posture Correction:**
Proper Sitting:
Use a chair with good lumbar support or place a small pillow behind your lower back.
Keep your feet flat on the floor or on a footrest.

Avoid crossing your legs as it can reduce circulation.

Standing Posture:

Stand up straight with your shoulders back and relaxed.

Distribute your weight evenly on both feet.

If standing for long periods, shift your weight from one foot to the other and take breaks to sit down.

Sleeping Position:

Sleep on your side, preferably the left side, to improve circulation to the heart and the baby.

Use a pregnancy pillow to support your belly and between your knees.

Avoid sleeping on your back as it can put pressure on the vena cava, a major blood vessel, and reduce blood flow.

2. Prenatal Yoga:

Prenatal yoga can improve flexibility, strength, and balance while reducing stress and anxiety.

Focus on gentle stretches and poses that open the hips and relieve back pain.

Walking:

Regular walking can improve circulation, boost energy levels, and promote better sleep.

Aim for at least 30 minutes of moderate walking most days of the week.

Swimming:

Swimming is a low-impact exercise that can relieve joint pain, reduce swelling, and improve cardiovascular health.

Water buoyancy supports your weight, reducing strain on your back and legs.

Nutrition:

1. Balanced Diet:

Eat a variety of fruits, vegetables, whole grains, lean proteins, and healthy fats.

Focus on nutrient-dense foods that provide essential vitamins and minerals for you and your baby.

Frequent Small Meals:

Eat small, frequent meals throughout the day to maintain steady blood sugar levels and prevent nausea.

Avoid large, heavy meals that can cause indigestion and heartburn.

Hydration:

Drink plenty of water throughout the day to stay hydrated and support overall health.
Proper hydration can help prevent constipation, reduce swelling, and improve energy levels.
Stress Management:

2. Relaxation Techniques:

Practice deep breathing exercises, meditation, or progressive muscle relaxation to reduce stress and promote relaxation.
Take a few minutes each day to sit quietly and focus on your breathing.
Time Management:
Prioritize tasks and delegate responsibilities to reduce feelings of overwhelm.
Take breaks throughout the day to rest and recharge.
Support System:
Lean on your support system, whether it's your partner, family, or friends, for emotional and practical support.
Join a prenatal support group to connect with other expectant mothers and share experiences.
Ergonomics:

3. Workplace Adjustments:

If you work at a desk, ensure your workstation is ergonomically set up to reduce strain on your body.
Use a chair with good back support and adjust the height so your feet are flat on the floor.
Household Tasks:
Avoid lifting heavy objects and ask for help with tasks that require bending or reaching.
Use tools and equipment that reduce strain, such as a step stool or a grabber.
Mental Well-being:

4. Positive Mindset:

Focus on the positive aspects of your pregnancy and the excitement of welcoming your baby.
Practice gratitude by keeping a journal of things you are thankful for each day.
Mindfulness:
Engage in mindfulness practices to stay present and reduce anxiety about the future.
Spend a few minutes each day in quiet reflection or guided meditation.
Counseling:
Consider speaking with a counselor or therapist if you experience significant stress, anxiety, or depression.
Prenatal counseling can provide tools and strategies to cope with emotional challenges.
By incorporating these lifestyle changes, you can effectively manage and alleviate many common pregnancy discomforts. Proper posture, regular exercise, balanced nutrition, stress

management, ergonomic adjustments, and mental well-being practices all contribute to a healthier and more comfortable pregnancy. Remember to consult with your healthcare provider before making significant changes to your routine, especially regarding exercise and diet.

While many pregnancy discomforts can be managed with lifestyle changes and natural remedies, certain symptoms may indicate more serious issues that require medical attention. Understanding when to seek help is crucial for the health and safety of both the mother and the baby.

5. Severe Abdominal Pain:

Possible Causes:

Severe abdominal pain can be a sign of various conditions, including preterm labor, placental abruption, or an ectopic pregnancy.

It can also indicate gastrointestinal issues like appendicitis or gallstones.

When to Seek Help:

If you experience sharp, severe, or persistent abdominal pain that doesn't go away after resting, contact your healthcare provider immediately.

Pain accompanied by other symptoms like fever, bleeding, or dizziness requires urgent medical evaluation.

6. Heavy Vaginal Bleeding:

Possible Causes:

Heavy bleeding can indicate miscarriage, placental abruption, or placenta previa.

Light spotting can be normal, but heavy bleeding is a cause for concern.

When to Seek Help:

Contact your healthcare provider immediately if you experience heavy bleeding, especially if it is accompanied by cramping or pain.

Any bleeding in the second or third trimester should be promptly evaluated.

7. Severe Headaches:

Possible Causes:

Severe headaches can be a sign of preeclampsia, a condition characterized by high blood pressure and protein in the urine.

They can also be caused by dehydration, stress, or migraines.

When to Seek Help:

Seek medical attention if you have a severe headache that doesn't go away with rest or medication, or if it's accompanied by vision changes, swelling, or upper abdominal pain. Report any sudden, severe headaches to your healthcare provider.

8. Swelling of the Hands and Face:

Possible Causes:

Swelling (edema) can be a normal part of pregnancy, but sudden or severe swelling can indicate preeclampsia.

When to Seek Help:

If you notice sudden or severe swelling in your hands, face, or around your eyes, contact your healthcare provider.

Swelling accompanied by other symptoms like headaches, vision changes, or abdominal pain requires immediate medical attention.

9. Persistent Vomiting:

Possible Causes:

Persistent vomiting can lead to dehydration and weight loss, conditions that require medical intervention.

It may indicate hyperemesis gravidarum, a severe form of morning sickness.

When to Seek Help:

Seek medical attention if you are unable to keep any food or fluids down for more than 24 hours.

Report persistent vomiting, especially if accompanied by weight loss or signs of dehydration (such as dark urine or dizziness).

10. Decreased Fetal Movement:

Possible Causes:

Decreased fetal movement can be a sign of fetal distress or other issues that need immediate evaluation.

When to Seek Help:

Contact your healthcare provider if you notice a significant decrease in your baby's movements or if you're unable to feel any movements over several hours.

Your provider may perform tests to ensure your baby's well-being.

11. High Fever:

Possible Causes:

A high fever can be a sign of an infection, which can be harmful to both mother and baby if not treated.

When to Seek Help:

Seek medical attention if you have a fever over 100.4°F (38°C) that doesn't respond to acetaminophen (Tylenol) or if it's accompanied by other symptoms like rash, headache, or abdominal pain.

12. **Difficulty Breathing or Chest Pain**:

Possible Causes:

Difficulty breathing or chest pain can indicate serious conditions such as pulmonary embolism, heart problems, or severe asthma.

When to Seek Help:

If you experience sudden or severe difficulty breathing, chest pain, or pressure, seek emergency medical attention immediately.

These symptoms can be life-threatening and require prompt evaluation and treatment.

13. **Signs of Preterm Labor:**

Possible Causes:

Preterm labor can occur before 37 weeks of pregnancy and can lead to premature birth if not managed properly.

When to Seek Help:

Contact your healthcare provider if you experience regular contractions, lower back pain, pelvic pressure, or changes in vaginal discharge (such as a watery, mucus-like, or bloody discharge) before 37 weeks.

Early intervention can help manage preterm labor and improve outcomes for you and your baby. By being aware of these warning signs and knowing when to seek medical attention, you can help ensure a safer and healthier pregnancy. Always trust your instincts and contact your healthcare provider if you have any concerns about your health or your baby's well-being. Prompt medical evaluation can address potential issues early and provide the necessary care and support.

As you journey through pregnancy, embracing the marvels and challenges it brings, remember that managing discomforts is not just about alleviating physical symptoms but also nurturing your emotional well-being. Each discomfort discussed in this chapter from morning sickness to insomnia is a testament to the unique journey of pregnancy. By understanding the causes, exploring relief measures, and implementing proactive strategies, you empower yourself to navigate these challenges with resilience and grace.

Through natural remedies, lifestyle adjustments, and knowing when to seek medical attention, you can safeguard your health and that of your baby. Moreover, prioritizing self-care practices for emotional well-being connecting with supportive relationships, practicing relaxation techniques, and engaging in gentle exercise fosters a positive mindset and enhances your pregnancy experience.

As you embark on this transformative path, trust in your body's ability to adapt and thrive. Seek guidance from healthcare providers, draw strength from your support system, and honor the journey as it unfolds. Remember, each discomfort conquered is a testament to your strength and the deep love you hold for your growing family.

May this chapter serve as a companion, offering insights and strategies to ensure a nourished and wholesome pregnancy. Embrace each moment, cherish the milestones, and celebrate the journey ahead with confidence and joy.

Chapter 8:

Special Considerations

Pregnancy is a transformative journey, one that brings immense joy and unique challenges. It's a time when your body requires extra care, attention, and nourishment to support both your health and the development of your baby. In Chapter 8, "Special Considerations," we delve into crucial aspects of pregnancy that demand special attention to ensure optimal wellness for both mother and baby.

This chapter is designed to guide you through the nuances of maintaining a healthy and balanced diet during pregnancy, managing health conditions, and navigating lifestyle changes. We'll start with "Safe Eating Practices," where you'll learn how to make informed food choices, avoid harmful substances, and maintain food safety to protect yourself and your growing baby. Following this, we address "Managing Health Conditions During Pregnancy," offering insights into handling common pregnancy-related conditions such as gestational diabetes, hypertension, and thyroid issues.

Our exploration continues with "Nutrition and Wellness," emphasizing the importance of mindful eating, maintaining a healthy gut microbiome, and safely incorporating medications and supplements. Lastly, we discuss "Lifestyle and Environmental Considerations," providing practical advice on managing travel, social gatherings, and environmental factors that may impact your pregnancy.

Each section is crafted to provide you with practical, science-backed advice and empathetic support, ensuring you feel empowered and confident in making the best choices for your health and your baby's well-being. By understanding and addressing these special considerations, you can navigate your pregnancy with greater ease and assurance, laying a strong foundation for a healthy, joyful motherhood journey.

Let's embark on this chapter together, equipping you with the knowledge and tools to nurture your body and baby through every stage of this incredible experience.

<u>Safe Eating Practices</u>

During pregnancy, maintaining safe eating practices is crucial to ensure the health and safety of both mother and baby. This involves being mindful of food choices, understanding which foods to avoid, and adhering to strict food safety measures.

Food Safety

Food safety becomes paramount during pregnancy due to the increased vulnerability to foodborne illnesses. Pregnant women are more susceptible to infections such as listeriosis and toxoplasmosis, which can have serious implications for both the mother and the developing baby.

Key Food Safety Tips:

- ❖ Wash Your Hands and Produce: Always wash your hands before and after handling food. Clean fruits and vegetables thoroughly to remove any potential contaminants.
- ❖ Cook Foods Thoroughly: Ensure that meats, poultry, seafood, and eggs are cooked to safe internal temperatures to kill harmful bacteria. Use a food thermometer to check doneness.
- ❖ Avoid Cross-Contamination: Use separate cutting boards for raw meats and vegetables. Clean all surfaces and utensils after use.
- ❖ Store Foods Properly: Refrigerate perishable foods promptly and keep your fridge at or below 40°F (4°C). Avoid consuming food past its expiration date.
- ❖ Avoid Unpasteurized Products: Steer clear of unpasteurized milk, cheese, and juices, as they can harbor harmful bacteria.
- ❖ Avoiding Harmful Foods
- ❖ Certain foods can pose risks during pregnancy due to potential contaminants or adverse effects on fetal development. Knowing which foods to avoid can help mitigate these risks.

Foods to Avoid:

Raw or Undercooked Seafood and Eggs: Sushi, sashimi, and raw shellfish can contain harmful bacteria and parasites. Similarly, raw eggs may harbor Salmonella.

High-Mercury Fish: Limit intake of high-mercury fish such as shark, swordfish, king mackerel, and tilefish. Opt for lower-mercury options like salmon, tilapia, and shrimp.

Deli Meats and Uncooked Hot Dogs: These can be contaminated with Listeria, which can cause serious infections. Reheat these foods until steaming hot before consuming.

Unpasteurized Dairy and Juices: Avoid unpasteurized milk, cheese (like brie and feta), and juices to reduce the risk of bacterial infections.

Raw Sprouts: Raw sprouts such as alfalfa, clover, and radish can be contaminated with E. coli or Salmonella.

Vegetarian and Vegan Pregnancy

A vegetarian or vegan diet can be healthy during pregnancy if well-planned to include all necessary nutrients. Special attention must be given to ensure adequate intake of key nutrients like protein, iron, vitamin B12, calcium, and omega-3 fatty acids.

Nutrient-Rich Vegetarian and Vegan Foods:

Protein: Incorporate a variety of protein sources such as beans, lentils, tofu, tempeh, nuts, seeds, and quinoa.

Iron: Include iron-rich foods like leafy greens, fortified cereals, lentils, and dried fruits. Pair these with vitamin C-rich foods to enhance absorption.

Vitamin B12: Since B12 is primarily found in animal products, consider fortified foods or supplements.

Calcium: Ensure sufficient calcium intake through fortified plant milks, leafy greens, tofu, and almonds.

Omega-3 Fatty Acids: Include sources like flaxseeds, chia seeds, walnuts, and algae-based supplements.

By adhering to these safe eating practices and being mindful of your dietary choices, you can support a healthy pregnancy and provide optimal nourishment for your growing baby.

Managing Health Conditions During Pregnancy

Pregnancy is a time of joy and anticipation, but it can also be a period of increased health challenges. Managing health conditions effectively during pregnancy is crucial for the well-being of both mother and baby. This section addresses common health conditions that may arise during pregnancy and offers guidance on how to manage them.

Gestational Diabetes Management

Gestational diabetes is a condition that develops during pregnancy and affects how your body uses sugar (glucose). It can lead to high blood sugar levels, which can affect your pregnancy and your baby's health. Managing gestational diabetes involves monitoring blood sugar levels, eating a healthy diet, and possibly taking medication.

Monitoring Blood Sugar Levels: Regular monitoring of blood glucose levels is essential. Your healthcare provider will guide you on how often to check your blood sugar and what your target levels should be.

Healthy Diet: A balanced diet that includes a variety of foods from all food groups is crucial. Focus on whole grains, fruits, vegetables, lean proteins, and healthy fats. Limiting sugary foods and refined carbohydrates can help keep blood sugar levels stable.

Physical Activity: Regular physical activity can help manage blood sugar levels. Discuss safe exercise options with your healthcare provider.

Medication: If diet and exercise aren't enough to control your blood sugar levels, your doctor may prescribe insulin or other medications.

Hypertension and Preeclampsia Management
High blood pressure (hypertension) and preeclampsia are serious conditions that can occur during pregnancy. Preeclampsia is characterized by high blood pressure and damage to other organs, often the liver and kidneys.

Regular Monitoring: Regular prenatal visits are essential to monitor your blood pressure and check for signs of preeclampsia.

Healthy Diet: A diet rich in fruits, vegetables, and whole grains, and low in sodium, can help manage blood pressure. Adequate hydration is also important.

Medication: Your healthcare provider may prescribe medication to control your blood pressure. It's crucial to take these medications as directed.

Rest and Stress Management: Rest and stress management techniques, such as prenatal yoga and meditation, can help lower blood pressure.

Thyroid Condition Management
Thyroid disorders, such as hypothyroidism (underactive thyroid) and hyperthyroidism (overactive thyroid), can affect pregnancy.

Regular Testing: Regular blood tests to monitor thyroid hormone levels are important. Your healthcare provider will determine the frequency of these tests.

Medication: Thyroid hormone replacement therapy or antithyroid medications may be necessary. It's essential to take these medications as prescribed and not skip doses.

Diet: A well-balanced diet that includes iodine-rich foods, such as fish, dairy, and iodized salt, can support thyroid function.

Autoimmune Disorder Management
Autoimmune disorders, such as lupus and rheumatoid arthritis, require special attention during pregnancy.

Medication Management: Work closely with your healthcare provider to manage medications. Some medications may need to be adjusted to ensure they are safe for pregnancy.

Monitoring: Regular monitoring of the condition and the health of the baby is essential. This may include more frequent prenatal visits and additional tests.

Lifestyle Adjustments: Maintaining a healthy lifestyle, including a balanced diet and regular physical activity, can help manage symptoms.

Managing health conditions during pregnancy requires collaboration with your healthcare provider. With careful monitoring and appropriate lifestyle adjustments, you can maintain your health and support the development of your baby.

Lifestyle and Environmental Considerations

During pregnancy, your lifestyle and environment play a significant role in your overall health and well-being. This section addresses important considerations, including safe travel practices, food safety, and navigating social gatherings.

Travel and Food Safety During Pregnancy
Traveling while pregnant can be enjoyable, but it's important to take certain precautions to ensure your safety and that of your baby.

Travel Tips:
Timing: The best time to travel is usually during the second trimester (14-28 weeks) when morning sickness has likely subsided and energy levels are higher.
Comfort: Wear comfortable clothing, take frequent breaks to stretch and walk, and stay hydrated.
Medical Care: Know the locations of medical facilities at your destination and carry a copy of your prenatal records.

Food Safety:
Safe Eating: Avoid foods that carry a higher risk of contamination, such as raw or undercooked seafood, unpasteurized dairy products, and deli meats. Always choose freshly prepared, fully cooked meals.
Water Safety: Drink bottled or purified water, especially when traveling to areas where water quality is questionable.
Hand Hygiene: Wash your hands frequently with soap and water, especially before eating.
Eating Out and Social Gatherings During Pregnancy
Navigating social events and eating out while pregnant requires mindfulness to maintain your nutritional needs and safety.

Choosing Safe Foods:
Restaurant Choices: Opt for restaurants known for their food safety practices. Avoid buffets and salad bars where food might be left out for long periods.
Menu Options: Select dishes that are cooked thoroughly. Avoid raw or undercooked meats, eggs, and fish.
Ask Questions: Don't hesitate to ask about ingredients and preparation methods to ensure they meet pregnancy safety standards.

Social Gatherings:
Buffet Tips: At gatherings, choose items from the buffet that are freshly prepared and kept at safe temperatures. Avoid foods that have been sitting out.
Bring Your Own: Consider bringing a dish that you know is safe to eat, ensuring you have at least one nutritious and safe option.
Alcohol Alternatives: Opt for non-alcoholic beverages such as sparkling water with a splash of fruit juice or mocktails to enjoy festive drinks without the risks.
Managing Social Pressures:

Stay Informed: Being knowledgeable about your dietary needs and restrictions can help you make informed choices and confidently decline unsafe foods.

Communicate: Share your dietary preferences and restrictions with hosts or dining companions to ensure there are safe options available.

Environmental Toxins and Pregnancy

Reducing exposure to environmental toxins is crucial for the health of both mother and baby.

Here are some key points to consider:

Household Products:

Cleaning Supplies: Choose non-toxic, natural cleaning products. Avoid harsh chemicals like ammonia, bleach, and certain solvents.

Personal Care Products: Opt for skincare and cosmetic products that are free from harmful chemicals such as parabens, phthalates, and synthetic fragrances.

Air Quality:

Ventilation: Ensure proper ventilation in your home, especially when using household cleaners or other chemicals.

Outdoor Air Quality: Stay indoors on days with poor air quality or high pollution levels. Use air purifiers to maintain clean indoor air.

Food and Water:

Pesticides: Choose organic produce when possible to reduce exposure to pesticides. Wash fruits and vegetables thoroughly.

Water: Use a water filter to remove potential contaminants from tap water.

Occupational Hazards:

Workplace Safety: If your job involves exposure to harmful substances, discuss with your employer about possible adjustments or protective measures to ensure a safe working environment.

By paying attention to lifestyle and environmental considerations, you can create a safer and healthier environment for both you and your baby. These steps will help you enjoy a more comfortable pregnancy while minimizing potential risks.

Navigating pregnancy involves making numerous adjustments to ensure the health and well-being of both mother and baby. This chapter on special considerations underscores the importance of adapting your lifestyle and environment to promote optimal outcomes during this crucial time.

Safe Eating Practices highlight the necessity of mindful food choices to avoid potential risks. Knowing which foods to avoid and practicing good food hygiene can significantly reduce the chances of foodborne illnesses. Whether you follow a traditional diet or are vegetarian or vegan, understanding the nutritional requirements and ensuring a balanced intake is vital.

Managing Health Conditions During Pregnancy emphasizes the importance of proactive healthcare. Conditions like gestational diabetes, hypertension, and thyroid disorders require special attention and management strategies to ensure a healthy pregnancy. Regular medical check-ups and following your healthcare provider's advice are crucial steps in managing these conditions effectively.

Nutrition and Wellness integrates mindful eating and the importance of a healthy gut microbiome. Maintaining balanced nutrition and understanding the role of supplements and medications can significantly enhance your well-being during pregnancy. This holistic approach supports both physical and mental health, ensuring a harmonious balance.

Lifestyle and Environmental Considerations provide practical advice on safe travel, food safety, and managing social gatherings. It also highlights the importance of reducing exposure to environmental toxins and creating a safe living environment. These measures collectively contribute to a healthier pregnancy experience.

As you move forward in your pregnancy journey, remember that every decision you make plays a role in nurturing your baby and yourself. Embrace these special considerations with confidence, knowing that you are making informed choices to support a healthy, joyful pregnancy. Celebrate each step of this journey, and cherish the unique experience of bringing new life into the world.

Chapter 9:

Postpartum Wellness

The journey of motherhood is an incredible, life-altering adventure that begins long before the birth of your child. It is a time filled with anticipation, joy, and sometimes, anxiety. The arrival of a new baby heralds a period of intense change not only in the dynamics of your family but also within your own body. Postpartum wellness is a crucial aspect of this transformative journey, focusing on the physical, nutritional, emotional, and mental health of new mothers. This chapter will delve into the critical phase following childbirth, offering practical guidance, expert advice, and a compassionate approach to ensure you navigate this period with confidence and grace.

In this chapter, we will explore five comprehensive sections designed to support your postpartum wellness. The first section, Physical Recovery, will address the healing process from childbirth and cesarean sections, managing postpartum pain and discomfort, and restoring core strength and pelvic floor health. Next, we will focus on Nutrition for Postpartum Wellness, emphasizing essential nutrients for lactation and breastfeeding, healthy meal planning and snack ideas, and the importance of hydration and electrolyte balance.

The third section, Weight Loss and Body Composition, will provide insights into safe and sustainable weight loss strategies, building lean muscle mass, and embracing body changes with self-acceptance. Following this, we will discuss Mental and Emotional Wellbeing, covering the management of postpartum depression and anxiety, building a support network and community, and prioritizing self-care and stress management. Finally, we will address Sleep and Rest, offering strategies for improving sleep with a new baby, the importance of rest and relaxation, and tips for napping and sleep training.

As you read through this chapter, remember that postpartum wellness is not a one-size-fits-all approach. Each mother's experience is unique, and it's essential to listen to your body, seek support when needed, and embrace this journey with patience and self-compassion. Whether you are a first-time mom or adding to your growing family, this chapter aims to be your supportive companion, guiding you towards enhanced health and wellbeing during this pivotal phase in your life.

Physical Recovery

Healing from Childbirth and Cesarean Sections

The postpartum period, often referred to as the "fourth trimester," is a critical time for a mother's body to heal and recover from the immense changes of pregnancy and childbirth. Healing from childbirth, whether it was a vaginal delivery or a cesarean section, involves various physical and emotional aspects.

For those who have experienced a vaginal delivery, the body undergoes significant stress and stretching. The perineum, the area between the vagina and anus, often requires healing due to tearing or episiotomy (a surgical cut made during delivery). Common symptoms in the immediate postpartum period include soreness, swelling, and bruising in this region. It is essential to keep the area clean and dry, using warm water to rinse after using the bathroom and avoiding harsh soaps or chemicals. Sitz baths, which involve sitting in warm water, can provide relief and promote healing.

For mothers who have undergone a cesarean section, the recovery process is different and can be more challenging due to the surgical nature of the birth. A cesarean section involves making an incision through the abdominal wall and uterus, which requires a longer healing time. Managing the incision site is crucial to prevent infection and promote healing. Keeping the area clean and dry, avoiding strenuous activities, and following the doctor's guidelines for wound care are essential steps. It is also important to monitor for any signs of infection, such as redness, swelling, or discharge, and to seek medical attention if needed.

Pain management is a significant aspect of postpartum recovery for both vaginal and cesarean deliveries. Over-the-counter pain relievers, such as ibuprofen or acetaminophen, can be effective for managing pain and discomfort. In some cases, doctors may prescribe stronger pain medications, especially for those recovering from a cesarean section. It is important to take these medications as prescribed and to communicate with your healthcare provider about any concerns or side effects.

Rest and proper nutrition are vital components of the healing process. The body requires additional calories and nutrients to repair tissues and regain strength. Consuming a balanced diet rich in protein, vitamins, and minerals can support the body's recovery. Hydration is also crucial, as it aids in healing and helps to alleviate common postpartum issues such as constipation.

Emotional healing is another important aspect of the postpartum period. The hormonal fluctuations that occur after childbirth can lead to mood swings, feelings of sadness, or anxiety.

It is essential to acknowledge these emotions and seek support from loved ones, healthcare providers, or support groups. Postpartum depression is a serious condition that affects many new mothers and requires professional attention and care.

Managing Postpartum Pain and Discomfort

The postpartum period is often accompanied by various forms of pain and discomfort, which can affect a new mother's ability to care for herself and her baby. Managing these symptoms effectively is crucial for promoting recovery and overall well-being.

One common source of postpartum pain is uterine contractions, also known as "afterpains." These contractions help the uterus return to its pre-pregnancy size and can be quite intense, especially during breastfeeding. Applying a warm compress to the lower abdomen or taking over-the-counter pain relief can help alleviate discomfort. Staying hydrated and emptying the bladder frequently can also reduce the severity of afterpains.

Breast engorgement is another source of discomfort for many new mothers. This condition occurs when the breasts become overly full with milk, leading to swelling, tenderness, and pain. To manage engorgement, it is essential to breastfeed frequently or express milk to relieve pressure. Applying cold compresses between feedings and warm compresses before breastfeeding can also provide relief. Wearing a supportive bra and avoiding tight clothing can help reduce discomfort.

Hemorrhoids and constipation are common postpartum issues, often resulting from the strain of childbirth or hormonal changes. To manage these symptoms, it is important to maintain a high-fiber diet, stay hydrated, and engage in gentle physical activity to promote regular bowel movements. Over-the-counter treatments, such as stool softeners or hemorrhoid creams, can also be effective. Sitz baths can provide relief for hemorrhoids by reducing swelling and discomfort.

For mothers recovering from a cesarean section, managing incision pain and discomfort is a significant aspect of the recovery process. Following the doctor's guidelines for wound care and taking prescribed pain medications as directed are essential steps. Gentle movements and avoiding heavy lifting or strenuous activities can prevent strain on the incision site. Using a pillow to support the abdomen while coughing, sneezing, or laughing can also help reduce discomfort.

Perinea pain and discomfort are common after a vaginal delivery, especially if there was tearing or an episiotomy. Using ice packs, sitz baths, and over-the-counter pain relief can help manage this discomfort. Keeping the perineal area clean and dry and wearing loose, breathable clothing can also promote healing and reduce irritation.

Fatigue is another common issue during the postpartum period. The demands of caring for a newborn, combined with the body's healing process, can lead to exhaustion. It is essential to prioritize rest and sleep whenever possible. Accepting help from family and friends, napping when the baby naps, and practicing relaxation techniques can all contribute to managing fatigue and promoting overall well-being.

Managing postpartum pain and discomfort involves a combination of physical care, pain relief strategies, and emotional support. It is important to communicate with healthcare providers about any persistent or severe pain and to seek medical advice when needed. By addressing these symptoms proactively, new mothers can support their recovery and focus on bonding with their baby.

Restoring Core Strength and Pelvic Floor Health
Restoring core strength and pelvic floor health is a vital aspect of postpartum recovery. Pregnancy and childbirth place significant strain on the abdominal muscles and pelvic floor, leading to weakness and potential issues such as diastasis recti, urinary incontinence, and pelvic organ prolapse. A targeted approach to rebuilding these areas can enhance overall physical health and prevent long-term complications.

Diastasis recti is a common condition where the abdominal muscles separate during pregnancy, creating a gap along the midline of the abdomen. This separation can lead to a weakened core, lower back pain, and a protruding belly. To address diastasis recti, it is essential to engage in exercises that strengthen the transverse abdominis, the deepest layer of abdominal muscles. Gentle exercises such as pelvic tilts, heel slides, and modified planks can help close the gap and restore core strength. It is important to avoid exercises that place excessive strain on the abdomen, such as traditional crunches or sit-ups, until the muscles have sufficiently healed.

The pelvic floor, a group of muscles that support the bladder, uterus, and bowel, undergoes significant stress during pregnancy and childbirth. Strengthening these muscles is crucial for preventing issues such as urinary incontinence and pelvic organ prolapse. Kegels exercises, which involve contracting and relaxing the pelvic floor muscles, are a simple and effective way to improve pelvic floor strength. Performing Kegels regularly, several times a day, can help restore muscle tone and function.

In addition to Kegel exercises, incorporating a variety of movements that engage the pelvic floor and core muscles can enhance overall strength and stability. Pilates and yoga are excellent options for postpartum exercise, as they focus on controlled movements and core engagement. These practices also promote relaxation and mental well-being, which are important aspects of postpartum recovery.

It is important to approach postpartum exercise gradually and to listen to your body. Starting with gentle activities such as walking or light stretching can help reintroduce physical activity without overloading the body. As strength and endurance improve, more challenging exercises can be incorporated. Consulting with a healthcare provider or a physical therapist specializing in postpartum recovery can provide personalized guidance and ensure that exercises are performed safely and effectively.

Maintaining proper posture and body mechanics is also essential for restoring core strength and pelvic floor health. Pregnancy often leads to changes in posture, with a tendency to arch the lower back and tilt the pelvis forward. Focusing on proper alignment and engaging the core muscles while performing daily activities, such as lifting the baby or carrying a diaper bag, can help protect the back and pelvic floor.

Nutrition plays a supportive role in muscle recovery and overall health. Consuming a balanced diet rich in protein, vitamins, and minerals provides the necessary building blocks for tissue repair and muscle growth. Hydration is also crucial, as it supports cellular function and aids in the body's recovery processes.

Restoring core strength and pelvic floor health is a multifaceted approach that involves targeted exercises, proper posture, gradual progression, and supportive nutrition. By prioritizing these aspects of physical recovery, new mothers can enhance their overall well-being, prevent long-term complications, and feel empowered in their postpartum journey.

Nutrition for Postpartum Wellness

Essential Nutrients for Lactation and Breastfeeding
Lactation and breastfeeding place increased nutritional demands on a new mother's body. Ensuring an adequate intake of essential nutrients is crucial for both the mother's health and the

baby's growth and development. Breast milk provides optimal nutrition for infants, containing the right balance of nutrients, antibodies, and beneficial compounds that support the baby's immune system and overall health.

Protein is a fundamental nutrient for lactating mothers, as it supports the production of breast milk and the repair of tissues. High-quality protein sources such as lean meats, poultry, fish, eggs, dairy products, legumes, nuts, and seeds should be incorporated into the diet. Aiming for a variety of protein sources ensures a diverse intake of amino acids, which are the building blocks of proteins.

Fats, particularly healthy fats, are essential for breastfeeding mothers. Omega-3 fatty acids, found in fatty fish like salmon and sardines, flaxseeds, chia seeds, and walnuts, play a crucial role in the development of the baby's brain and nervous system. Including sources of healthy fats such as avocados, olive oil, and nuts in the diet supports both maternal and infant health.

Carbohydrates are the body's primary source of energy and are important for sustaining energy levels during lactation. Choosing complex carbohydrates such as whole grains, fruits, vegetables, and legumes provides a steady release of energy and essential nutrients like fiber, vitamins, and minerals. Fiber is particularly important for preventing constipation, a common issue during the postpartum period.

Calcium is a vital mineral for lactating mothers, as it is crucial for the development of the baby's bones and teeth. Dairy products, fortified plant-based milk, leafy green vegetables, and almonds are excellent sources of calcium. Adequate calcium intake also supports the mother's bone health, preventing the depletion of calcium stores during breastfeeding.

Iron is another essential nutrient for postpartum wellness, as it supports the production of red blood cells and prevents anemia. Iron-rich foods include lean meats, poultry, fish, beans, lentils, tofu, and fortified cereals. Consuming vitamin C-rich foods like citrus fruits, strawberries, and bell peppers alongside iron sources enhances iron absorption.

Vitamin D plays a crucial role in bone health and immune function. Sun exposure is a natural source of vitamin D, but dietary sources such as fatty fish, fortified dairy products, and egg yolks are also important. In some cases, a vitamin D supplement may be recommended, especially for those with limited sun exposure.

B vitamins, including B12, B6, and folate, are essential for energy production, brain function, and the formation of red blood cells. Animal products, such as meat, poultry, fish, eggs, and dairy, are primary sources of B12, while B6 and folate can be found in whole grains, leafy green vegetables, legumes, and fortified cereals.

Hydration is another critical aspect of nutrition for lactation. Breastfeeding mothers require additional fluids to produce breast milk and maintain overall hydration. Drinking water regularly throughout the day, consuming hydrating foods like fruits and vegetables, and avoiding excessive caffeine or sugary beverages can help meet hydration needs.

A balanced and nutrient-dense diet is essential for supporting lactation and breastfeeding. By prioritizing a variety of whole foods, staying hydrated, and considering potential supplementation, new mothers can ensure they meet their nutritional needs and support their baby's growth and development.

Healthy Meal Planning and Snack Ideas
Healthy meal planning and snacking are important aspects of postpartum nutrition. With the demands of caring for a newborn, having quick and nutritious meal options can make a significant difference in maintaining energy levels and overall wellness.

Start by planning meals that are balanced and rich in essential nutrients. Incorporate a variety of protein sources, healthy fats, complex carbohydrates, and plenty of fruits and vegetables. Preparing meals in advance and utilizing batch cooking can save time and reduce stress. Consider making large portions of soups, stews, casseroles, or grain salads that can be easily reheated and enjoyed over several days.

Breakfast is an important meal to kick start the day with energy and nutrients. Options like oatmeal topped with fresh fruit and nuts, Greek yogurt with honey and granola, or a smoothie made with spinach, banana, and protein powder can provide a nutritious start. Including protein and fiber in the morning helps keep hunger at bay and supports sustained energy levels.

Lunch and dinner should focus on balanced meals that include a source of protein, vegetables, and whole grains. Grilled chicken or fish with quinoa and roasted vegetables, lentil soup with a side salad, or a hearty grain bowl with chickpeas, avocado, and mixed greens are nutritious and satisfying options. Incorporating a variety of herbs and spices can enhance flavor and provide additional health benefits.

Snacking is an essential part of postpartum nutrition, as it helps maintain energy levels throughout the day. Healthy snack options include fresh fruit, vegetable sticks with hummus, nuts and seeds, whole-grain crackers with cheese, or a piece of whole fruit with nut butter. Keeping nutritious snacks readily available can help avoid reaching for less healthy options when hunger strikes.

Hydration is also key, and incorporating hydrating foods and beverages can support overall well-being. Infused water with slices of cucumber and mint, herbal teas, or coconut water are refreshing options. Including water-rich fruits and vegetables, such as watermelon, cucumber, and oranges, can also contribute to hydration.

Creating a meal plan for the week can streamline grocery shopping and meal preparation. Consider dedicating time once a week to plan meals, make a shopping list, and prep ingredients. This approach not only saves time but also ensures that nutritious options are always on hand.

In summary, healthy meal planning and snacking involve incorporating a variety of nutrient-dense foods, preparing meals in advance, and keeping nutritious snacks available. By prioritizing balanced meals and staying hydrated, new mothers can support their postpartum recovery and overall well-being.

Hydration and Electrolyte Balance
Hydration is a crucial aspect of postpartum wellness, particularly for breastfeeding mothers. Adequate fluid intake is necessary to support the production of breast milk, maintain energy levels, and promote overall health. Understanding the importance of hydration and electrolyte balance can help new mothers meet their needs effectively.

Water is the primary component of breast milk, and breastfeeding mothers require additional fluids to produce milk and stay hydrated. Drinking water regularly throughout the day is essential, and it is helpful to keep a water bottle nearby as a reminder to drink frequently. Listening to the body's thirst signals and drinking when thirsty is a good practice, but it is also beneficial to aim for a baseline intake of about 8-12 cups of fluids per day.

In addition to water, other hydrating beverages can contribute to fluid intake. Herbal teas, such as chamomile or peppermint, can be soothing and hydrating. Coconut water is an excellent source of natural electrolytes and can be a refreshing alternative to sugary drinks. Avoiding excessive caffeine and sugary beverages is important, as they can lead to dehydration and energy crashes.

Electrolytes, such as sodium, potassium, and magnesium, play a vital role in maintaining fluid balance and supporting muscle and nerve function. Consuming a variety of foods rich in electrolytes can help maintain this balance. Bananas, avocados, leafy green vegetables, nuts, seeds, and dairy products are excellent sources of these essential minerals.

For mothers experiencing heavy sweating or frequent urination, such as during the summer months or when engaging in physical activity, replenishing electrolytes becomes even more important. Including electrolyte-rich foods in the diet and considering electrolyte-enhanced beverages, like sports drinks with low sugar content or electrolyte tablets, can help maintain optimal balance.

Dehydration can have negative effects on both the mother and the baby. For the mother, it can lead to fatigue, headaches, dizziness, and decreased milk supply. For the baby, inadequate hydration in the mother can result in lower milk production and potential feeding difficulties. Therefore, prioritizing hydration is essential for both maternal and infant health.

Hydration and electrolyte balance are critical components of postpartum wellness. By drinking plenty of water, incorporating hydrating beverages, and consuming electrolyte-rich foods, new mothers can support their body's needs and promote optimal health for themselves and their babies.

Weight Loss and Body Composition

Safe and Sustainable Weight Loss Strategies
Postpartum weight loss is a common goal for many new mothers, but it is essential to approach this process with patience, self-compassion, and a focus on health rather than quick results. Safe and sustainable weight loss strategies can help new mothers regain their pre-pregnancy weight and improve their overall well-being without compromising their health or the health of their baby.

The first step in postpartum weight loss is to set realistic and achievable goals. It is important to remember that it took nine months to gain the pregnancy weight, and it is natural for it to take several months to lose it. Setting small, incremental goals can make the process more manageable and less overwhelming. Celebrating each milestone, no matter how small, can also help maintain motivation.

A balanced and nutritious diet is a cornerstone of sustainable weight loss. Focusing on whole foods, such as fruits, vegetables, lean proteins, whole grains, and healthy fats, provides the body with the necessary nutrients while promoting satiety and energy. Avoiding restrictive diets or extreme calorie cutting is important, as these approaches can lead to nutrient deficiencies, decreased milk supply, and other health issues.

Portion control is a practical strategy for managing calorie intake without feeling deprived. Using smaller plates, paying attention to hunger and fullness cues, and eating mindfully can help prevent overeating. Snacking on nutrient-dense foods and avoiding empty-calorie snacks like chips, cookies, and sugary beverages can also support weight loss efforts.

Physical activity is another key component of postpartum weight loss. Engaging in regular exercise helps burn calories, build muscle, and improve overall fitness. Low-impact activities, such as walking, swimming, and postpartum yoga, are gentle on the body and can be gradually increased in intensity as the mother's strength and endurance improve. Strength training exercises, such as bodyweight exercises, resistance bands, or light weights, can help build lean muscle mass, which boosts metabolism and aids in weight loss.

Breastfeeding can also support postpartum weight loss. Producing breast milk burns extra calories, and many mothers find that breastfeeding helps them shed pregnancy weight more quickly. However, it is important to ensure that weight loss does not negatively impact milk supply. Eating enough to maintain energy levels and meet the demands of breastfeeding is crucial.

Getting adequate sleep is often challenging for new mothers, but it plays a significant role in weight loss. Sleep deprivation can affect hormones that regulate hunger and satiety, leading to increased cravings and overeating. Prioritizing rest whenever possible, even through short naps, can support weight loss efforts.

Stress management is another important aspect of postpartum weight loss. Chronic stress can lead to emotional eating and hinder weight loss progress. Incorporating stress-reducing activities, such as mindfulness meditation, deep breathing exercises, or spending time outdoors, can help manage stress levels and support overall well-being.

In conclusion, safe and sustainable weight loss strategies for postpartum mothers involve setting realistic goals, focusing on a balanced diet, incorporating regular physical activity, and managing stress and sleep. By taking a gradual and holistic approach, new mothers can achieve their weight loss goals while prioritizing their health and the health of their baby.

Building Lean Muscle Mass
Building lean muscle mass is an important aspect of postpartum wellness and body composition. Lean muscle not only helps in weight management by increasing metabolism but also improves overall strength, energy levels, and functional fitness, which are crucial for the daily demands of motherhood.

Starting with gentle exercises is key for new mothers, especially in the initial postpartum period when the body is still healing. Once given the all-clear by a healthcare provider, incorporating strength training exercises can help rebuild muscle mass and strength. Bodyweight exercises, such as squats, lunges, push-ups, and planks, are excellent starting points. These exercises engage multiple muscle groups and can be modified to match the mother's fitness level.

Progression is important in strength training. Gradually increasing the intensity, frequency, and resistance of exercises helps to continually challenge the muscles and promote growth. Resistance bands, light weights, and kettlebells can be introduced to add resistance as strength improves. It's essential to focus on proper form and technique to prevent injury and ensure that the exercises effectively target the intended muscle groups.

Core exercises are particularly important for new mothers, as the core muscles often weaken during pregnancy. Strengthening the core can help alleviate postpartum back pain, improve posture, and restore stability. Gentle core exercises such as pelvic tilts, bridges, and abdominal bracing can be gradually progressed to more challenging movements like planks and side planks.

In addition to structured exercise, incorporating more movement into daily life can contribute to muscle building. Activities such as carrying the baby, using a stroller for brisk walks, doing household chores, or playing with older children all provide opportunities to engage and strengthen muscles.

Nutrition plays a crucial role in muscle building. Adequate protein intake is essential for muscle repair and growth. Including a source of protein in each meal and snack, such as lean meats, fish, eggs, dairy, legumes, nuts, and seeds, supports muscle recovery. Additionally, consuming a balanced diet with sufficient carbohydrates and healthy fats provides the necessary energy for exercise and daily activities.

Hydration is also vital for muscle function and recovery. Drinking plenty of water before, during, and after workouts helps maintain muscle function and prevents dehydration, which can impair performance and recovery.

Recovery is a critical component of muscle building. Ensuring adequate rest and allowing time for muscles to repair and grow is essential. This means incorporating rest days into the workout routine and listening to the body to avoid overtraining, which can lead to injury and hinder progress.

Building lean muscle mass postpartum is a gradual process that requires consistency, patience, and a balanced approach. By focusing on progressive strength training, incorporating more movement into daily life, ensuring proper nutrition and hydration, and prioritizing recovery, new mothers can effectively rebuild muscle strength and enhance their overall health and well-being.

Navigating Body Changes with Self-Acceptance
The postpartum period brings about significant physical changes, and navigating these changes with self-acceptance is crucial for overall well-being. Embracing the postpartum body with compassion and understanding can positively impact mental and emotional health, fostering a positive self-image and confidence.

It's important to recognize that every mother's postpartum journey is unique, and there is no "right" way to look after childbirth. Comparing oneself to others, especially in the age of social media, can be detrimental. Instead, focusing on personal progress and celebrating the body's incredible ability to grow and nurture a new life can cultivate a sense of gratitude and respect for one's body.

Body positivity and self-acceptance start with changing the internal dialogue. Replacing negative self-talk with positive affirmations can shift the mindset towards a more supportive and loving perspective. Reminding oneself of the strength, resilience, and beauty of the postpartum body can reinforce positive feelings and reduce self-criticism.

Setting realistic expectations is key. The body undergoes significant changes during pregnancy and childbirth, and it takes time to recover. Recognizing that the postpartum body may never look exactly the same as it did pre-pregnancy is important. Embracing these changes as part of the journey and celebrating the new version of oneself can foster self-acceptance.

Focusing on health and well-being rather than appearance can shift the emphasis from weight and shape to overall wellness. Engaging in physical activities that are enjoyable and make the body feel good, eating nutritious foods that nourish and energize, and prioritizing self-care practices that support mental and emotional health all contribute to a positive body image.

Support from loved ones can also play a significant role in navigating body changes. Sharing feelings and experiences with a partner, friends, or a support group can provide validation and encouragement. Surrounding oneself with positive influences and avoiding those that perpetuate unrealistic body standards can help maintain a healthy perspective.

Professional support, such as counseling or therapy, can be beneficial for those struggling with body image issues. A mental health professional can provide tools and strategies to cope with negative thoughts and foster self-acceptance.

In conclusion, navigating postpartum body changes with self-acceptance involves embracing the body's new reality with compassion, focusing on health and well-being, and seeking support when needed. By cultivating a positive mindset and prioritizing self-care, new mothers can develop a healthy and loving relationship with their postpartum bodies, enhancing their overall wellness and confidence.

Mental and Emotional Wellbeing
Managing Postpartum Depression and Anxiety
The postpartum period can be a vulnerable time for new mothers, with significant changes in hormones, lifestyle, and responsibilities. Managing postpartum depression (PPD) and anxiety is crucial for both the mother's and the baby's health. Understanding the signs, seeking appropriate help, and implementing effective coping strategies can make a significant difference.

Postpartum depression is more than just the "baby blues," which are common and usually resolve within a couple of weeks. PPD is a more severe and persistent form of depression that can occur anytime within the first year after childbirth. Symptoms of PPD can include intense sadness, feelings of hopelessness, loss of interest in activities, changes in appetite or sleep patterns, fatigue, and difficulty bonding with the baby, and thoughts of self-harm or harming the baby.

Postpartum anxiety, on the other hand, can manifest as excessive worry, irritability, and restlessness, physical symptoms like rapid heartbeat or dizziness, and intrusive thoughts. Both

PPD and postpartum anxiety require attention and treatment, as they can impact the mother's ability to care for herself and her baby.

Recognizing the signs of PPD and anxiety is the first step towards managing them. It's important for new mothers to monitor their mental health and be honest about their feelings. If symptoms persist for more than two weeks, interfere with daily functioning, or cause distress, seeking professional help is essential. Healthcare providers, such as obstetricians, midwives, or mental health specialists, can provide appropriate support and treatment options.

Treatment for PPD and anxiety can include therapy, medication, or a combination of both. Cognitive-behavioral therapy (CBT) and interpersonal therapy (IPT) are effective forms of therapy that can help mothers understand and manage their thoughts, feelings, and behaviors. In some cases, antidepressant or anti-anxiety medications may be prescribed to alleviate symptoms.

Building a Support Network and Community
Building a strong support network and community is essential for the mental and emotional well-being of new mothers. The postpartum period can be overwhelming and isolating, but with a robust support system, mothers can navigate these challenges more effectively and feel less alone in their journey.

A support network begins with immediate family and friends. Partners play a critical role, providing emotional support, practical assistance, and sharing the responsibilities of childcare. Open communication with a partner about needs, feelings, and expectations is crucial. Partners should be encouraged to actively participate in the baby's care and household tasks, ensuring that the mother has time to rest and recuperate.

Extended family members, such as parents, siblings, or in-laws, can also offer valuable support. They can help with tasks like cooking, cleaning, or babysitting, allowing the new mother to focus on her recovery and bonding with the baby. It's important for mothers to communicate their needs clearly and accept help when offered.

Friends can be a source of emotional support and companionship. Regular check-ins, whether through phone calls, video chats, or in-person visits, can help new mothers feel connected and supported. Friends who are also parents can offer empathy, understanding, and practical advice based on their own experiences.

Support groups specifically for new mothers can be incredibly beneficial. These groups provide a safe space for mothers to share their experiences, challenges, and successes. Hearing from others who are going through similar situations can be reassuring and help normalize the ups and downs of motherhood. Many communities offer in-person support groups through hospitals, community centers, or parenting organizations. Online support groups and forums can also be valuable, offering flexibility and the opportunity to connect with a diverse group of mothers.

Professional support should not be overlooked. Healthcare providers, such as obstetricians, midwives, and pediatricians, can offer guidance on physical and emotional health. Mental health professionals, including therapists and counselors, can provide specialized support for managing postpartum depression, anxiety, or other emotional challenges. Lactation consultants can assist with breastfeeding issues, ensuring that both mother and baby are thriving.

Engaging in community activities can help new mothers feel connected and less isolated. Parenting classes, baby-and-me fitness classes, or local playgroups provide opportunities to meet other parents and form new friendships. Community resources, such as libraries or recreational centers, often offer programs and events for families, creating additional avenues for social interaction and support.

Technology can also play a role in building a support network. Social media platforms, parenting apps, and online communities can help mothers stay connected, access information, and find support. However, it's important to use technology mindfully and avoid comparing oneself to the often idealized portrayals of motherhood seen online.

Self-advocacy is a crucial component of building a support network. New mothers should feel empowered to ask for help and set boundaries to protect their well-being. This might involve saying no to certain requests, delegating tasks, or scheduling time for self-care. Recognizing that it is okay to need and accept help is vital for mental and emotional health.
Building a support network and community is a key aspect of postpartum wellness. By connecting with family, friends, support groups, and professionals, new mothers can create a strong foundation of support that helps them navigate the challenges of the postpartum period. Embracing this network can enhance emotional resilience, reduce feelings of isolation, and foster a positive and nurturing environment for both mother and baby.

<u>Prioritizing Self-Care and Stress Management</u>

Prioritizing self-care and managing stress are fundamental to maintaining mental and emotional well-being during the postpartum period. New mothers often face numerous demands, and it can be easy to overlook their own needs. However, taking time for self-care is essential for their overall health and ability to care for their baby.

Self-Care involves engaging in activities that nourish the body, mind, and spirit. It's important for new mothers to identify what self-care means to them and incorporate these practices into their daily routine. Self-care can take many forms, from physical activities and relaxation techniques to hobbies and social interactions.

Physical self-care is vital. Engaging in regular exercise, even if it's just a short walk, can boost mood, energy levels, and overall well-being. Postpartum yoga or gentle stretching can help relieve tension and promote relaxation. Adequate nutrition and hydration are also crucial components of physical self-care. Eating a balanced diet rich in fruits, vegetables, whole grains, and lean proteins supports recovery and energy levels.

Relaxation techniques can help manage stress and promote mental clarity. Mindfulness meditation, deep breathing exercises, and progressive muscle relaxation are effective ways to reduce stress and anxiety. Setting aside time each day, even if it's just a few minutes, to practice these techniques can make a significant difference in a new mother's stress levels.

Engaging in hobbies and activities that bring joy and relaxation is another important aspect of self-care. Whether it's reading, crafting, gardening, or listening to music, finding time for enjoyable activities can provide a much-needed mental break and enhance emotional well-being.

Social self-care involves nurturing relationships and maintaining social connections. Spending time with friends and family, joining support groups, or participating in community activities can provide emotional support and reduce feelings of isolation. It's important for new mothers to communicate their needs and set boundaries with others to ensure they are receiving the support they need.

Professional self-care includes seeking support from healthcare providers, therapists, or counselors. Regular check-ups with a healthcare provider can ensure physical health is on track, while therapy or counseling can provide additional support for mental and emotional health.

Sleep is a critical component of self-care, yet it is often disrupted for new mothers. Prioritizing rest whenever possible, even through short naps, can help manage fatigue and improve overall well-being. Establishing a sleep routine, asking for help with nighttime feedings, and creating a restful sleep environment can support better sleep.

Setting realistic expectations and being kind to oneself are important elements of self-care. The postpartum period is a time of adjustment, and it's normal to feel overwhelmed. Recognizing that it's okay to ask for help, take breaks, and prioritize self-care can reduce stress and improve overall health.

Prioritizing self-care and managing stress are essential for the mental and emotional well-being of new mothers. By engaging in physical, relaxation, social, and professional self-care practices, new mothers can enhance their resilience, reduce stress, and foster a positive and healthy postpartum experience. Embracing self-care not only benefits the mother but also creates a nurturing environment for the baby.

Sleep and Rest

Strategies for Improving Sleep with a New Baby
Sleep can be elusive for new mothers, but finding strategies to improve sleep with a new baby is crucial for overall health and well-being. Although the demands of a newborn can make uninterrupted sleep challenging, there are ways to maximize the quality and quantity of rest.

Establishing a bedtime routine can signal to both the mother and the baby that it's time to wind down. This routine might include activities such as a warm bath, gentle massage, reading a book, or singing a lullaby. Creating a calm and soothing environment can help the baby settle more easily and promote better sleep for both mother and child.

Sleep when the baby sleeps is a common piece of advice for new mothers, and it's valuable to take naps during the day whenever the baby naps. Even short naps can help reduce fatigue and improve alertness. While it might be tempting to use the baby's nap time for household chores or other tasks, prioritizing sleep can be more beneficial in the long run.

Sharing nighttime responsibilities with a partner can help ensure that both parents get some rest. Taking turns feeding, changing, and soothing the baby can prevent one parent from becoming overly sleep-deprived. If breastfeeding, mothers can pump milk so the partner can handle some feedings.

Creating a sleep-friendly environment is important for both mother and baby. Keeping the bedroom cool, dark, and quiet can promote better sleep. Using white noise machines, blackout curtains, and comfortable bedding can make the sleep environment more conducive to rest.

Safe co-sleeping arrangements, such as using a bedside bassinet, can make nighttime feedings easier and less disruptive. This arrangement allows the baby to be close by while ensuring a safe sleep environment. It's important to follow safe sleep guidelines to reduce the risk of Sudden Infant Death Syndrome (SIDS).

Limiting caffeine intake, especially in the afternoon and evening, can help improve sleep quality. While it's tempting to rely on caffeine to combat daytime fatigue, excessive intake can interfere with the ability to fall and stay asleep.

Practicing relaxation techniques before bed can help calm the mind and prepare for sleep. Mindfulness meditation, deep breathing exercises, or gentle yoga can reduce stress and promote relaxation. Avoiding screens and electronic devices at least an hour before bed can also improve sleep quality, as the blue light emitted from screens can interfere with the production of melatonin, the sleep hormone.

Adjusting expectations around sleep can help reduce frustration. Newborns typically wake frequently, and it's normal for sleep patterns to be irregular in the early months. Understanding that sleep will gradually improve can help new mothers feel more patient and less stressed about nighttime awakenings.

The Importance of Rest and Relaxation
Rest and relaxation are vital components of postpartum wellness, often overlooked amid the whirlwind of new motherhood. Rest is essential not only for physical recovery but also for mental and emotional well-being. Emphasizing the importance of rest and finding ways to incorporate relaxation into daily routines can significantly enhance a new mother's overall health and ability to care for her baby.

Physical rest is crucial for the body's recovery after childbirth. Pregnancy and delivery, whether vaginal or cesarean, place significant demands on the body. Rest allows the body to heal and regain strength. This includes not only sleep but also taking breaks from strenuous activities and avoiding overexertion. Mothers should be encouraged to listen to their bodies and rest when needed, without feeling guilty or pressured to resume normal activities too quickly.

Mental and emotional rest are equally important. The postpartum period is a time of emotional highs and lows, and it's essential to find moments of calm and relaxation to recharge mentally. Taking time for activities that provide emotional relief, such as reading, listening to music, or engaging in a hobby, can help reduce stress and improve mood.

Relaxation techniques can be particularly beneficial for new mothers. Practices such as mindfulness meditation, deep breathing exercises, and progressive muscle relaxation can help manage stress and promote a sense of calm. These techniques can be easily integrated into daily routines, providing quick and effective ways to relax.

Setting boundaries and learning to say no is an important aspect of prioritizing rest. New mothers often face numerous demands from family, friends, and social obligations. It's essential to recognize the importance of rest and protect time for it. This might involve delegating tasks, asking for help, or simply saying no to certain requests.

Creating a restful environment can support relaxation and improve the quality of rest. This includes ensuring the bedroom is a comfortable, sleep-friendly space and minimizing disruptions during rest periods. Incorporating calming elements, such as soft lighting, soothing scents, or relaxing sounds, can enhance the environment's ability to promote rest.

Engaging in restorative activities can also contribute to relaxation. Gentle exercises, such as yoga or tai chi, can promote physical relaxation and mental clarity. Warm baths, massages, and other self-care practices can help soothe the body and mind. Finding time for these activities, even in small increments, can make a significant difference in overall well-being.

Partners and family members play a crucial role in supporting a new mother's need for rest. They can help by taking on more responsibilities, providing practical assistance, and encouraging the mother to take breaks. Open communication about the importance of rest and the need for support can help ensure that mothers receive the rest they need.

Incorporating moments of rest throughout the day can also be beneficial. Short breaks, even if just a few minutes, can provide a mental and physical reset. Techniques such as the Pomodoro Technique, which involves working in short bursts with regular breaks, can help manage tasks without feeling overwhelmed.

Rest and relaxation are essential for postpartum wellness. By prioritizing rest, engaging in relaxation techniques, and creating a supportive environment, new mothers can enhance their physical, mental, and emotional health. Emphasizing the importance of rest and finding practical ways to incorporate it into daily routines can significantly improve the postpartum experience, leading to a healthier and happier mother and baby.

Tips for Napping and Sleep Training

Napping and sleep training are practical strategies that can help new mothers manage their sleep needs and establish healthy sleep habits for their babies. While every baby is different, and sleep patterns can vary, these tips can provide a foundation for improving sleep quality for both mother and child.

Napping Tips for New Mothers:

Sleep When the Baby Sleeps: This is one of the most common pieces of advice for new mothers and for good reason. Taking naps when the baby naps can help compensate for the fragmented nighttime sleep. Even short naps can reduce fatigue and boost energy levels.

Create a Sleep-Conducive Environment: Ensure that the nap environment is quiet, dark, and cool. Use blackout curtains, white noise machines, or earplugs to minimize disruptions. A comfortable sleeping area can make it easier to fall asleep quickly and improve the quality of rest.

Limit Caffeine Intake: Reducing caffeine consumption, especially in the afternoon and evening, can improve the ability to nap and the overall quality of sleep. Opt for decaffeinated beverages or herbal teas as alternatives.

Practice Relaxation Techniques: Engage in activities that promote relaxation before napping, such as deep breathing exercises, mindfulness meditation, or gentle stretching. These techniques can help calm the mind and prepare the body for rest.

Set Realistic Expectations: Understand that naps may not always be possible, especially during busy days. When napping isn't feasible, taking short breaks to relax and unwind can still provide some benefits.

Sleep Training Tips for Babies:

Establish a Consistent Bedtime Routine: A predictable bedtime routine can signal to the baby that it's time to sleep. Activities such as a warm bath, gentle massage, feeding, and reading a story can create a calming pre-sleep ritual.

Create a Sleep-Friendly Environment: Ensure the baby's sleep area is safe, comfortable, and conducive to sleep. This includes a firm mattress, breathable bedding, a cool room temperature, and minimal noise and light.

Follow a Flexible Schedule: While it's important to have a routine, being flexible with the baby's sleep schedule can help accommodate their natural sleep patterns. Pay attention to the baby's sleep cues, such as yawning, rubbing eyes, or fussiness, and adjust the schedule as needed.

Teach Self-Soothing Techniques: Encouraging the baby to self-soothe can help them fall asleep independently. This might involve allowing the baby to settle themselves to sleep after being placed in the crib drowsy but awake, or using a comforting object like a pacifier or a soft blanket.

Gradually Reduce Night Feedings: As the baby grows, they may need fewer nighttime feedings. Gradually reducing the frequency and duration of night feedings can help the baby sleep for longer stretches. Consult with a pediatrician to determine when it's appropriate to start this process.

Be Patient and Consistent: Sleep training takes time and consistency. It's important to remain patient and stay consistent with the chosen approach, even if progress seems slow. Every baby is different, and it may take time to establish healthy sleep habits.

Support for Mothers During Sleep Training:

Seek Support and Advice: Don't hesitate to seek support and advice from healthcare providers, lactation consultants, or sleep coaches. They can offer personalized guidance and address specific concerns related to sleep training.

Share Responsibilities with a Partner: Involving a partner in the sleep training process can provide additional support and make the experience less stressful. Partners can take turns soothing the baby, handling nighttime feedings, and participating in bedtime routines.

Practice Self-Care: During the sleep training period, it's important for mothers to prioritize self-care. This includes taking breaks, engaging in relaxing activities, and seeking emotional support when needed. Self-care can help manage the stress and exhaustion that often accompany sleep training.

Join Support Groups: Connecting with other mothers who are going through similar experiences can provide emotional support and practical tips. Support groups, both in-person and online, offer a sense of community and understanding.

Incorporating napping and sleep training strategies can help new mothers manage their sleep needs and establish healthy sleep habits for their babies. By following practical tips and seeking support, mothers can improve the quality of sleep for both themselves and their children, leading to a more restful and balanced postpartum experience.

With this, we conclude the chapter on Postpartum Wellness, hoping it will guide you through your journey towards enhanced health and well-being during this pivotal phase in your life.